W0228137

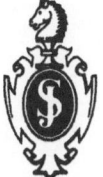

Fundamental Anatomy for Operative Orthopaedic Surgery is the second of a number of atlas-texts describing the essential anatomical basis of a range of common surgical procedures. Safe surgery is founded upon careful dissection and clear identification of vital structures. Knowledge of the appropriate anatomy and anatomical relations is therefore essential, not only during surgical training, but as the cornerstone of surgical practice. In this book clear line diagrams facing each page of text illustrate the important features that have to be identified.

Already published:

– General Surgery

Other titles planned include:

– Obstetrics and Gynaecology
– Cardiothoracic Surgery
– Plastic and Reconstructive Surgery
– Urology
– Neurosurgery

S.T. Donell and A.W.F. Lettin

Fundamental Anatomy for Operative Orthopaedic Surgery

With 121 Figures
drawn by Danielle G. Konyn

Springer-Verlag
London Berlin Heidelberg New York
Paris Tokyo Hong Kong

S. T. Donell, BSc, FRCS
Senior Orthopaedic Registrar, Institute of Orthopaedics at the Middlesex
Hospital, Mortimer Street, London WC1, UK

A. W. F. Lettin, MS, FRCS
Consultant Orthopaedic Surgeon, Royal National Orthopaedic Hospital,
London WC1, UK

ISBN 978-3-540-19669-3   ISBN 978-1-4471-1850-3 (eBook)
DOI 10.1007/978-1-4471-1850-3

British Library Cataloguing in Publication Data
Donell, S. T. (Simon Thomas) 1956–
  Fundamental anatomy for operative orthopaedic surgery.
  1. Humans. Anatomy
  I. Title II. Lettin, A. W. F. 1931–
  611
  ISBN 978-3-540-19669-3

Library of Congress Cataloging-in Publication-Data
Donell, S. T. (Simon Thomas), 1956–
  Fundamental anatomy for operative orthopaedic surgery /
  S. T. Donell, A. W. F. Lettin.
  p. sm. — (Fundamental anatomy)
  ISBN 978-3-540-19669-3
  1. Orthopedic surgery—At lases.   2. Anatomy, Surgical and topographical—
At lases.   3. Orthopedics.   I. Lettin, A. W. F. (Alan W. F.)   II. Title.   III. Series.
  [DNLM: 1. Anatomy.   QS 4 D681f]
  RD733.2.D66   1991
  617.3—dc20
  DNLM/DLC   91–4609
  for Library of Congress   CIP

Typeset by Wilmaset, Birkenhead, Wirral

28/3830–543210 Printed on acid-free paper

Preface

A sound knowledge of anatomy remains the basis of safe surgery. However, the detailed descriptive anatomy which was learnt and frequently forgotten is giving way to a more practical approach directed towards the needs of the surgeon.

Most orthopaedic operations are carried out on the bones and joints. Orthopaedic surgery is therefore largely the surgery of exposure of these structures. This book, which is one of a series, describes the important anatomical structures which are encountered in approaches used in orthopaedic surgery. Each approach, or part of an approach, may be used for a variety of operations.

In this book the illustrations of the limbs are all of the right side. The transverse sections are viewed from above.

This book is not meant to be a substitute for a textbook of systematic anatomy but rather an aide-memoire for the surgeon in training to use before entering the operating theatre or examination halls. We hope it will be of value for those preparing for the new Basic Science, Clinical Surgery and Specialist Orthopaedic examinations of the Royal Surgical Colleges.

1991   S.T.D.
                                                                        A.W.F.L.

Contents

Glossary

A	Anconeus	FCR	Flexor carpi radialis
	Artery	FCU	Flexor carpi ulnaris
AbdDV	Abductor digiti quinti	FDB	Flexor digitorum brevis
AbdH	Abductor hallucis	FDL	Flexor digitorum longus
AbPL	Abductor pollicis longus	FDP	Flexor digitorum profundus
ACL	Anterior cruciate ligament	FDS	Flexor digitorum sublimis
AddH	Adductor hallucis	FDV	Flexor digiti quinti
A–T	Achilles tendon	FHB	Flexor hallucis brevis
B	Biceps	FHL	Flexor hallucis longus
BF	Biceps femoris	FPL	Flexor pollicis longus
B–R	Brachioradialis	GM	Gluteus medius
C–B	Coracobrachialis	IVC	Inferior vena cava
ECR	Extensor carpi radialis	LG	Lateral gastrocnemius
ECRB	Extensor carpi radialis brevis	MG	Medial gastrocnemius
		N	Nerve
ECRL	Extensor carpi radialis longus	PB	Peroneus brevis
		PCL	Posterior cruciate ligament
ECU	Extensor carpi ulnaris	PL	Palmaris longus
EDB	Extensor digitorum brevis		Peroneus longus
EDC	Extensor digitorum communis	PM	Pectoralis major
		PT	Peroneus tertius
EDL	Extensor digitorum longus		Pronator teres
EDmin	Extensor digiti minimi	S–M	Semimembranosus
EH	Extensor hallucis	S–T	Semitendinosus
EHB	Extensor hallucis brevis	T	Tibia
EHL	Extensor hallucis longus	TA	Tibialis anterior
EPB	Extensor pollicis brevis	TP	Tibialis posterior
EPL	Extensor pollicis longus	V	Vein
F	Fibula	VL	Vastus lateralis

I. Upper Limb

Approach to the Brachial Plexus

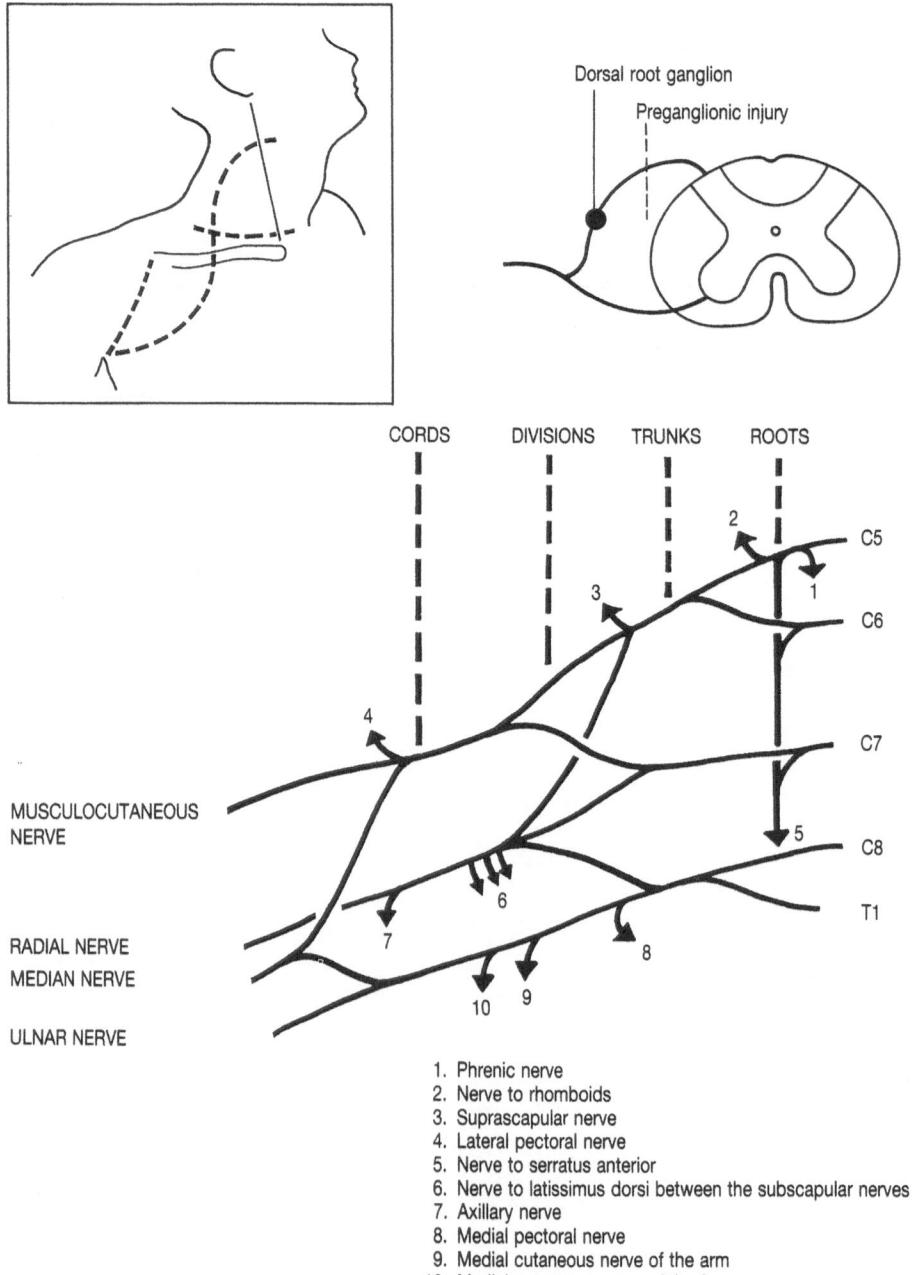

Dorsal root ganglion

Preganglionic injury

CORDS   DIVISIONS   TRUNKS   ROOTS

C5
C6
C7
C8
T1

MUSCULOCUTANEOUS NERVE

RADIAL NERVE
MEDIAN NERVE

ULNAR NERVE

1. Phrenic nerve
2. Nerve to rhomboids
3. Suprascapular nerve
4. Lateral pectoral nerve
5. Nerve to serratus anterior
6. Nerve to latissimus dorsi between the subscapular nerves
7. Axillary nerve
8. Medial pectoral nerve
9. Medial cutaneous nerve of the arm
10. Medial cutaneous nerve of the forearm

Fig. a. Diagram of the brachial plexus.

The brachial plexus may be damaged in open, or closed injuries, or damaged during operations on the root of the neck and then be amenable to repair. The majority of injuries are due to great violence and result in traction on the nerve roots. If the site of rupture is preganglionic then it is not amenable to repair.

The plexus is made up of 5 roots, which form 3 trunks, dividing into 6 divisions, which reform into 3 cords (Fig. a). The detailed anatomy is variable, but by careful clinical examination it is possible to localise the level of injury. For instance, in upper plexus injuries, if the serratus anterior muscle is working then the injury must be distal to the C5 nerve root.

The radial nerve supplies all the extensor muscles of the upper limb and sensation to the back of the hand. The musculocutaneous nerve supplies the elbow flexors, biceps, brachialis, and coracobrachialis, as well as sensation to the lateral side of the forearm. The median nerve supplies all the forearm flexors, except flexor carpi ulnaris and the ulnar half of flexor digitorum profundus, as well as the muscles of the thenar eminence, and sensation to the radial three and a half digits. The ulnar nerve supplies, in addition to the flexor carpi ulnaris and half of flexor digitorum profundus, all the small muscles of the hand, except the thenar muscles, and sensation to the ulnar one and a half digits.

Approach to the Brachial Plexus (continued)

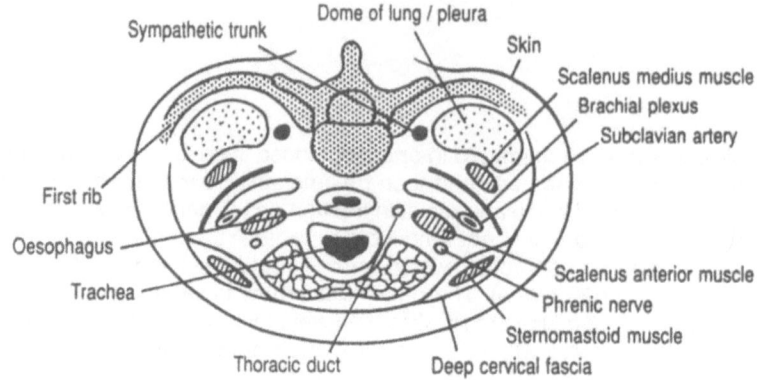

Sympathetic trunk
Dome of lung / pleura
Skin
Scalenus medius muscle
Brachial plexus
Subclavian artery
First rib
Oesophagus
Trachea
Scalenus anterior muscle
Phrenic nerve
Sternomastoid muscle
Thoracic duct
Deep cervical fascia

Fig. b. Transverse section through the root of the neck.

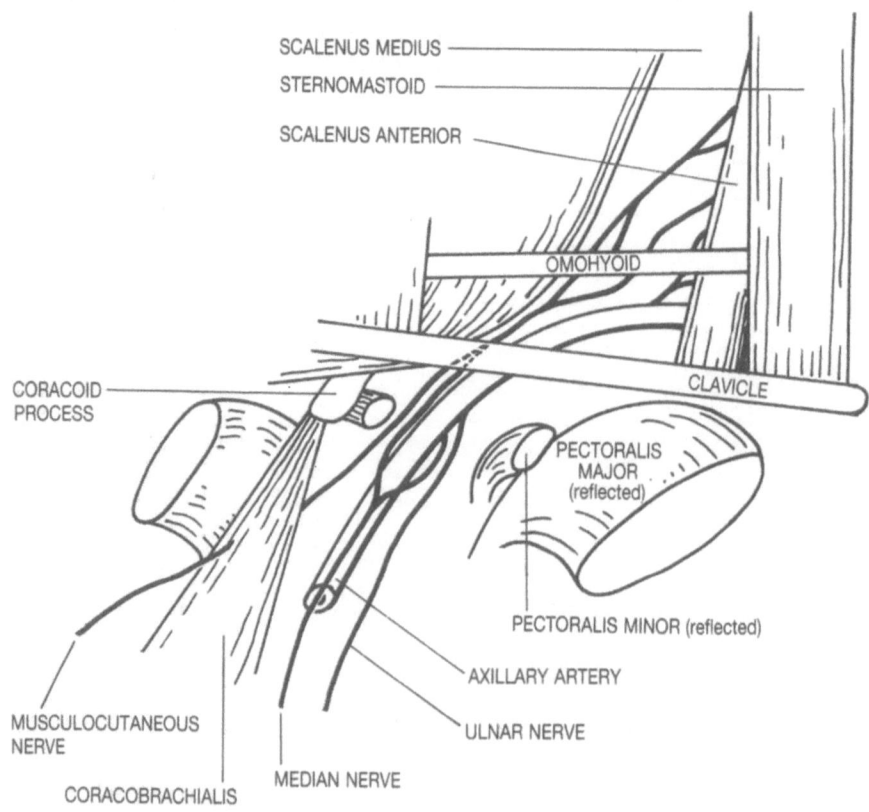

SCALENUS MEDIUS
STERNOMASTOID
SCALENUS ANTERIOR
OMOHYOID
CLAVICLE
CORACOID PROCESS
PECTORALIS MAJOR (reflected)
PECTORALIS MINOR (reflected)
AXILLARY ARTERY
ULNAR NERVE
MUSCULOCUTANEOUS NERVE
MEDIAN NERVE
CORACOBRACHIALIS

Fig. c. Anterior view of the relations of the brachial plexus.

Usually the upper trunk or the lower trunk alone needs to be explored. If the whole plexus needs to be exposed excise the middle third of the clavicle.

Exposure above the Clavicle

- Identify and excise the external jugular vein and the transverse cervical vessels to gain access to the deeper structures.

- Identify the omohyoid muscle which is cordlike. The brachial plexus lies immediately deep to it.

- The pulsatile internal jugular vein lies in the deep angle between the sternomastoid and scalenus anterior.

- To gain access to the lower trunk, detach scalenus anterior close to its insertion into the first rib. Avoid damaging the phrenic nerve, and the thoracic duct in left-sided operations (Fig. b).

Exposure below the Clavicle

- Divide and reflect medially pectoralis major to gain access to the deeper structures. Pectoralis minor may also be divided at its insertion to the coracoid (Fig. c). Take care to preserve their nerve supply, the medial and lateral pectoral nerves.

Approaches to the Shoulder

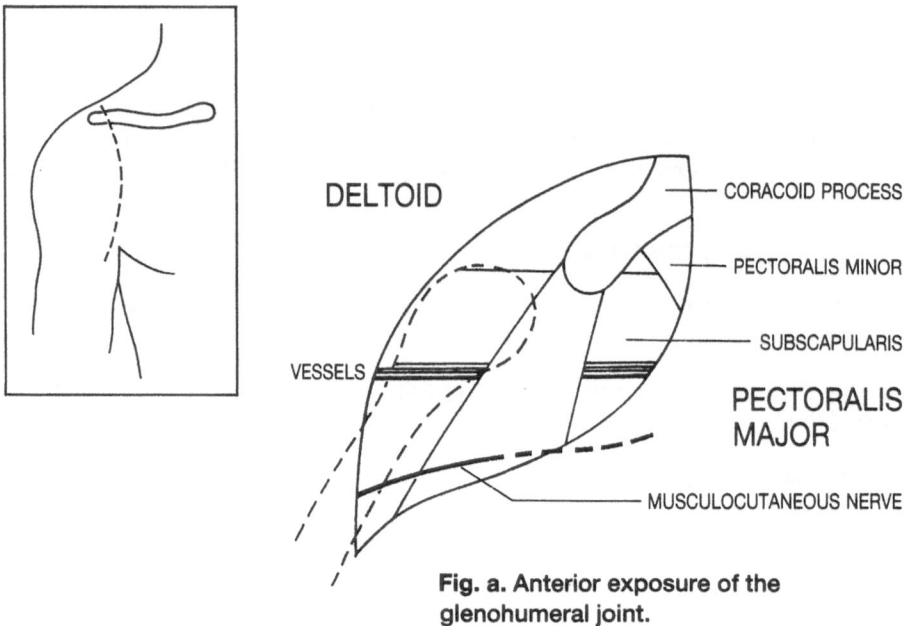

Fig. a. Anterior exposure of the glenohumeral joint.

DELTOID

VESSELS

CORACOID PROCESS

PECTORALIS MINOR

SUBSCAPULARIS

PECTORALIS MAJOR

MUSCULOCUTANEOUS NERVE

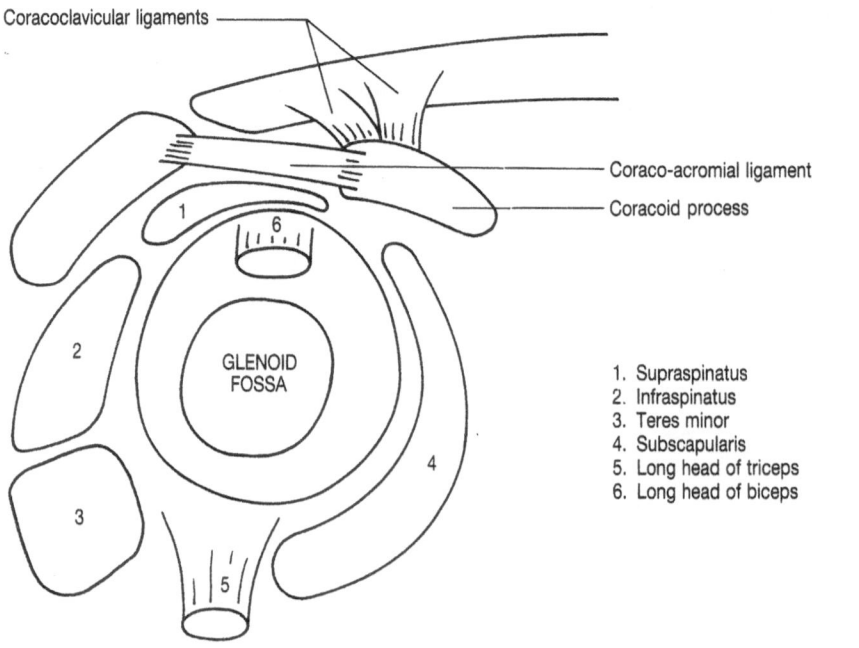

Coracoclavicular ligaments

Coraco-acromial ligament

Coracoid process

GLENOID FOSSA

1. Supraspinatus
2. Infraspinatus
3. Teres minor
4. Subscapularis
5. Long head of triceps
6. Long head of biceps

Fig. b. The shoulder joint.

The glenohumeral joint lies obliquely on the thoracic cage. The glenoid fossa is anteverted 30° and the humeral head is retroverted 60°. This is important in siting a humeral prosthesis to avoid dislocation.

Anterior

This exposure is used for repairing recurrent anterior dislocation, and also for joint arthroplasty, and the treatment of fractures of the neck of the humerus.

- Identify the deltopectoral groove. Ligate and excise the cephalic vein and coagulate its tributaries. Separate the deltoid from pectoralis major along the whole length of the deltopectoral groove.

- Perform an osteotomy of the tip of the coracoid process, or divide coracobrachialis and short head of biceps close to their origin to expose subscapularis (Fig. a). Avoid damage to the musculocutaneous nerve as it pierces coracobrachialis in the distal part of the wound.

- Divide subscapularis vertically at its musculotendinous junction to expose the capsule of the joint.

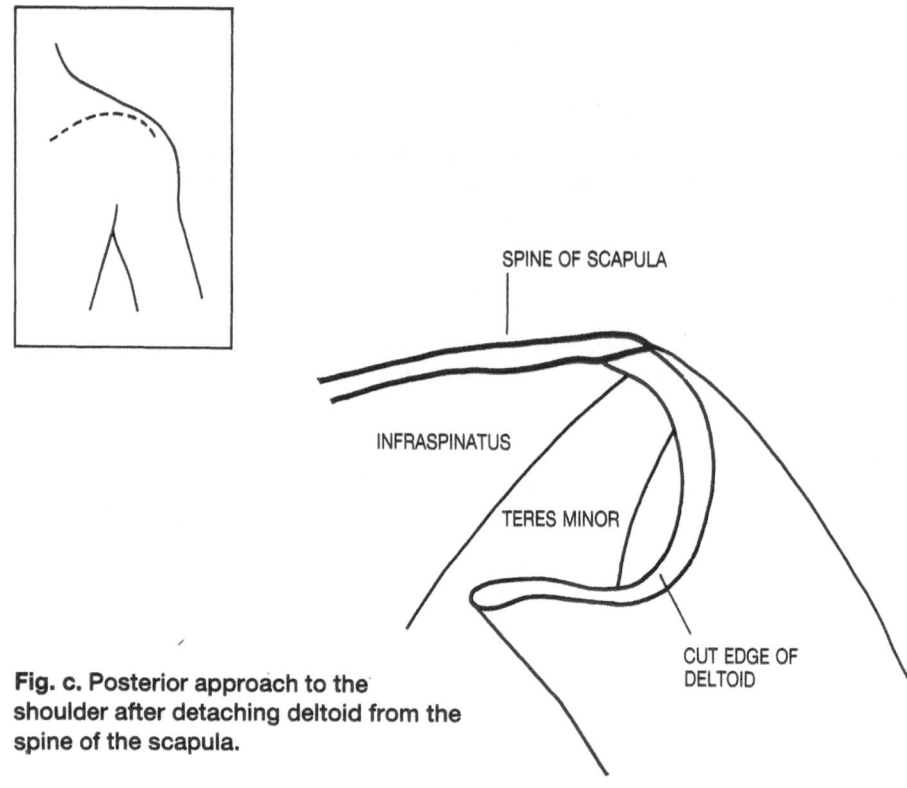

Fig. c. Posterior approach to the shoulder after detaching deltoid from the spine of the scapula.

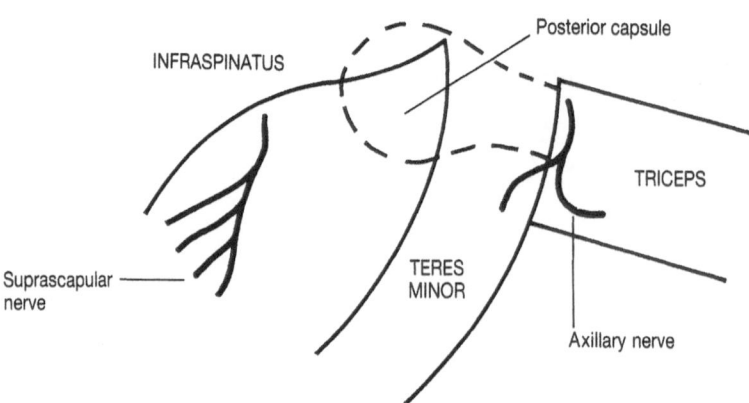

Fig. d. Posterior capsule of the shoulder exposed.

Posterior

This is used in recurrent posterior dislocations, and in shoulder arthrodesis.

- Deepen the wound by detaching deltoid from the spine of the scapula and reflect it laterally (Fig. c).

- Separate teres minor and infraspinatus to expose the capsule. Note the axillary and suprascapular nerves on either side of the operative field (Fig. d).

Approaches to the Shoulder (continued)

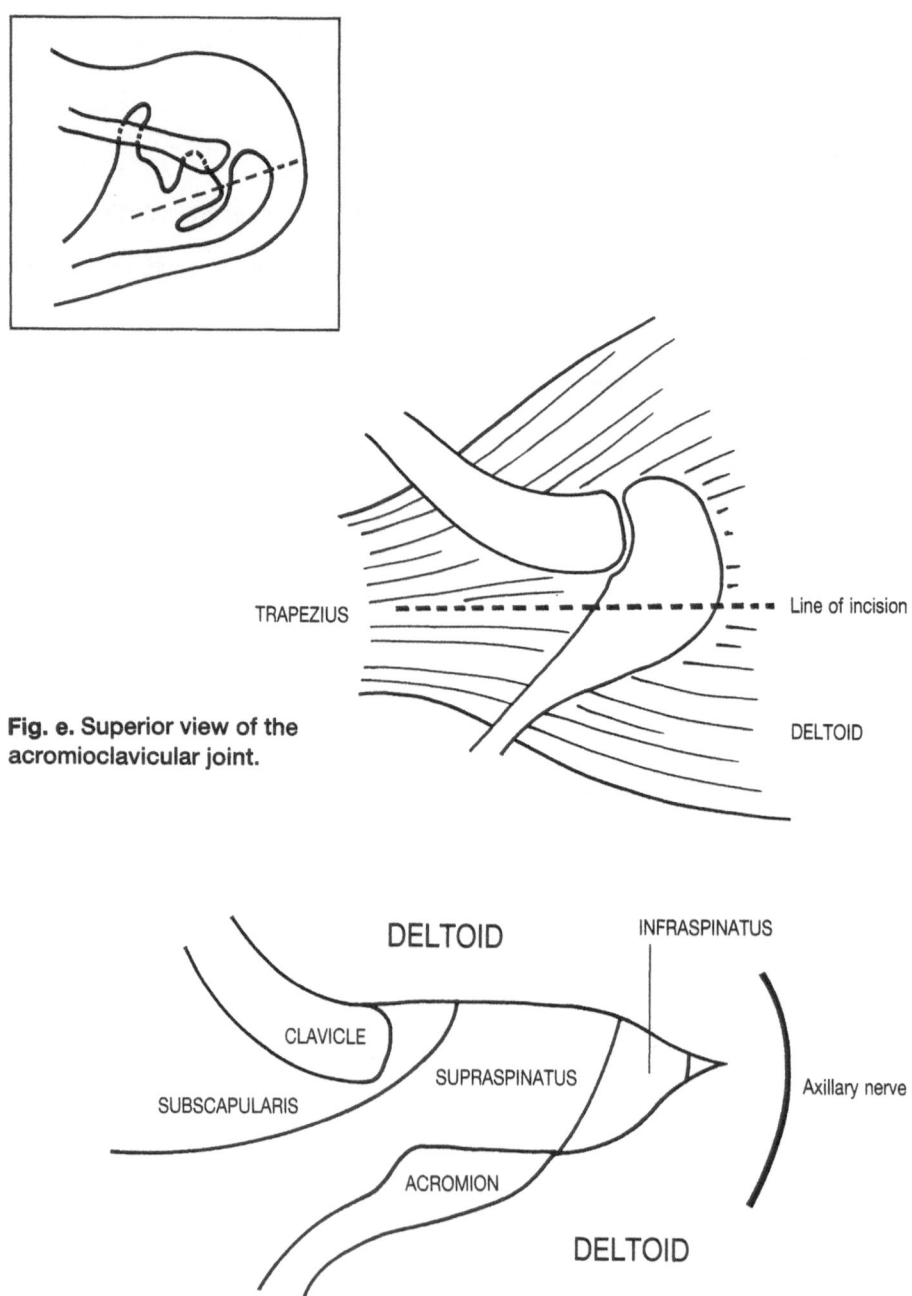

Fig. e. Superior view of the acromioclavicular joint.

TRAPEZIUS

Line of incision

DELTOID

DELTOID

INFRASPINATUS

CLAVICLE

SUPRASPINATUS

Axillary nerve

SUBSCAPULARIS

ACROMION

DELTOID

Fig. f. Superior view of the rotator cuff.

Transacromial

This is used to expose the rotator cuff (supraspinatus, infraspinatus, and teres minor) when there is a major tear (Fig. b, page 6).

- Deepen the wound by splitting trapezius in the line of its fibres and dividing the intervening acromion (Fig. e). If necessary gain greater access by excising the anterior acromion (Fig. f).

- Split the fibres of deltoid to no more than 3 cm to avoid damage to the axillary nerve as it wraps around the surgical neck of the humerus deep to deltoid.

Approaches to the Humerus

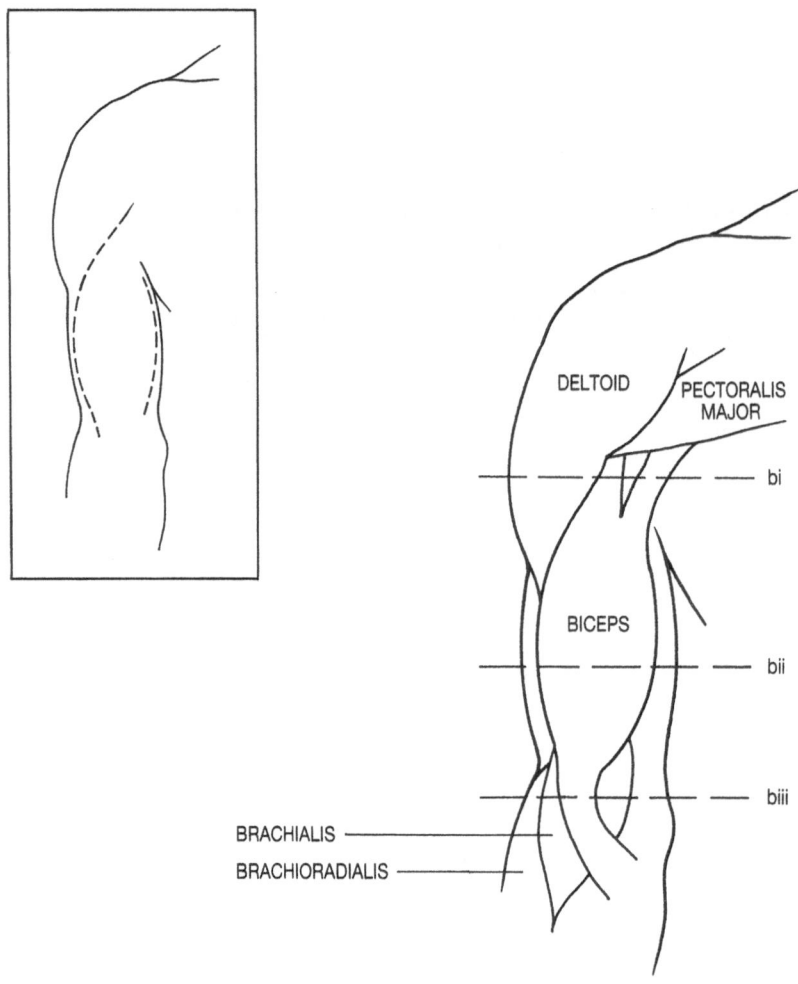

Fig. a. Anterior view of the muscles of the upper arm.

DELTOID

PECTORALIS MAJOR

bi

BICEPS

bii

biii

BRACHIALIS

BRACHIORADIALIS

The neurovascular structures apart from the radial nerve lie on the medial side of the humerus.

Anterolateral

All or part of the incision can be used as necessary.

- Expose the proximal third of the shaft through the deltopectoral groove as for the anterior shoulder approach and then divide the humeral attachment of pectoralis major (Fig. a).

- Identify coracobrachialis as it lies deep to biceps and detach it subperiosteally from the anteromedial aspect of the humerus (Fig. b i).

- Expose the distal two-thirds of the humerus by splitting the lateral part of brachialis. The radial nerve spirals round the humerus in the radial groove and is protected by the lateral part of brachialis (Fig. b ii).

Approaches to the Humerus (continued)

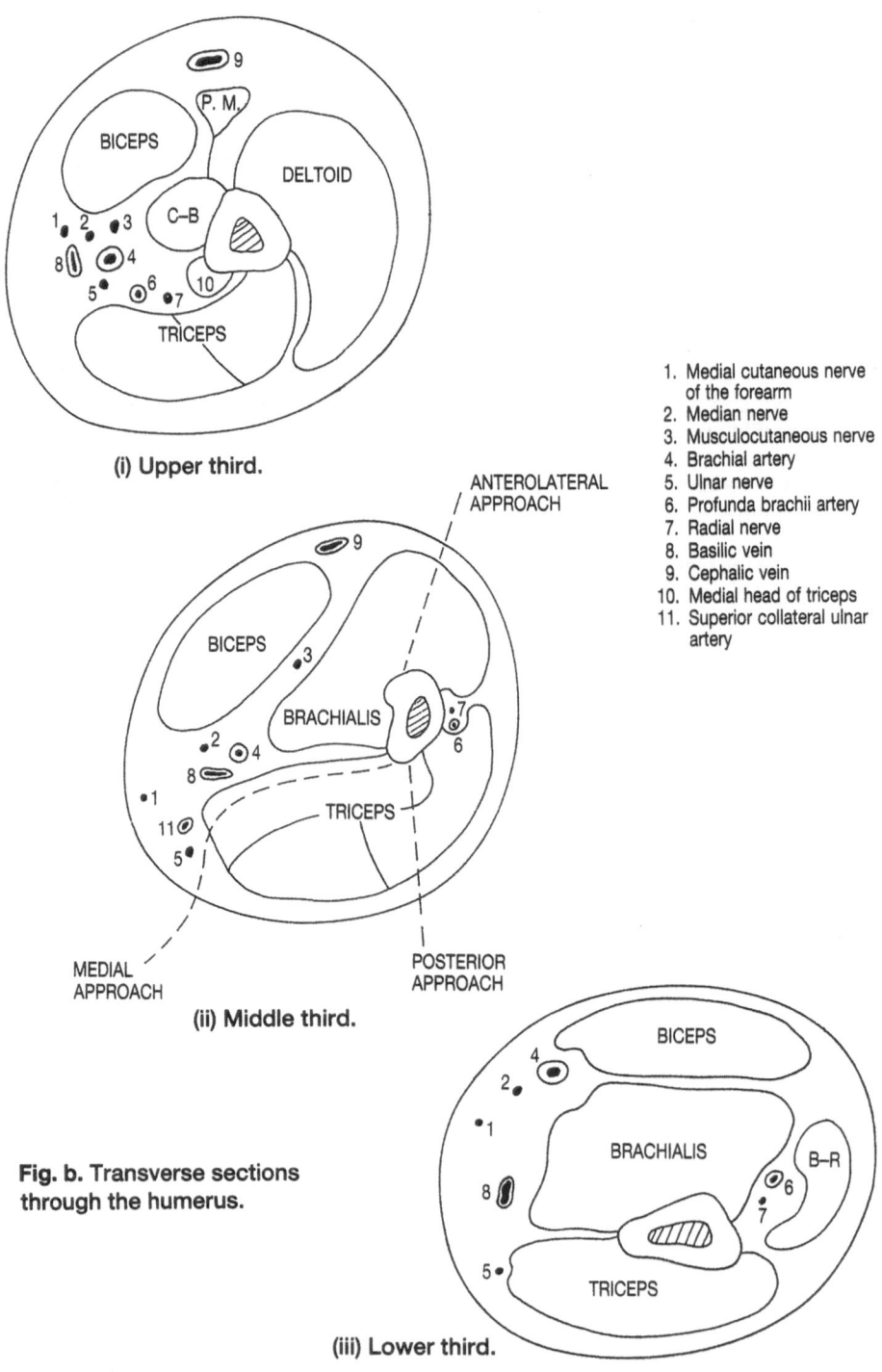

(i) Upper third.

1. Medial cutaneous nerve of the forearm
2. Median nerve
3. Musculocutaneous nerve
4. Brachial artery
5. Ulnar nerve
6. Profunda brachii artery
7. Radial nerve
8. Basilic vein
9. Cephalic vein
10. Medial head of triceps
11. Superior collateral ulnar artery

ANTEROLATERAL / APPROACH

MEDIAL APPROACH

POSTERIOR APPROACH

(ii) Middle third.

Fig. b. Transverse sections through the humerus.

(iii) Lower third.

Posterior

The incision is vertical in the midline of the arm. This approach exposes the middle and distal thirds of the shaft and can be extended into the elbow. It is used for fixing fractures of the humeral shaft.

- Expose the bone by incising through triceps (Fig. b ii).

- The radial nerve is at risk as it crosses the posterior aspect of the humerus from medially to laterally in the proximal part of the wound and also laterally as it lies deep to brachioradialis in the distal part of the wound (Fig. b iii).

Medial

- Expose the distal humerus by freeing the ulnar nerve from the triceps and approach the bone behind the intermuscular septum (Fig. b).

- When exposing the shaft more proximally avoid damage to the radial nerve.

Approaches to the Elbow

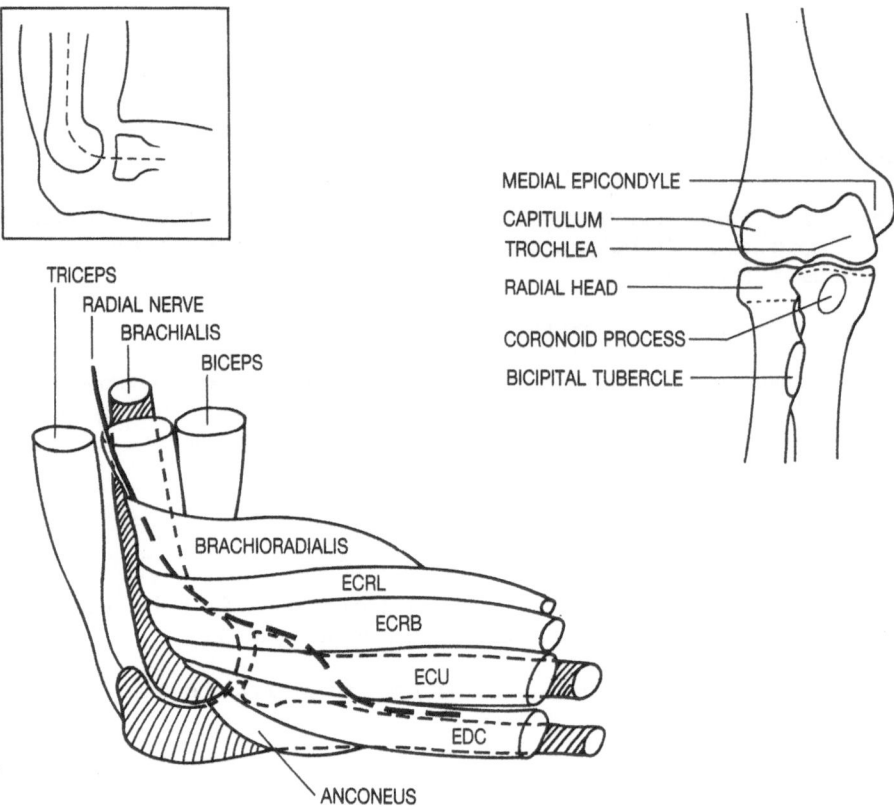

MEDIAL EPICONDYLE
CAPITULUM
TROCHLEA
RADIAL HEAD
CORONOID PROCESS
BICIPITAL TUBERCLE

TRICEPS
RADIAL NERVE
BRACHIALIS
BICEPS

BRACHIORADIALIS
ECRL
ECRB
ECU
EDC
ANCONEUS

Fig. a. Lateral view of the elbow.

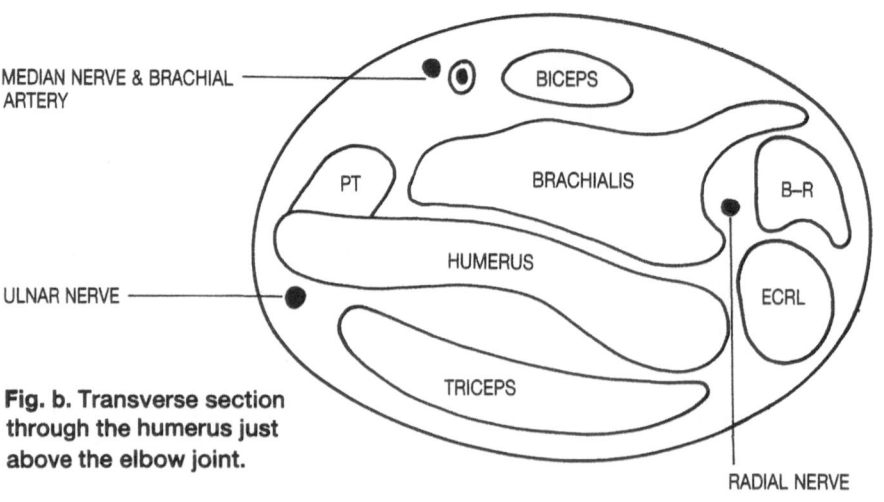

MEDIAN NERVE & BRACHIAL ARTERY

BICEPS

PT

BRACHIALIS

B–R

HUMERUS

ECRL

ULNAR NERVE

TRICEPS

Fig. b. Transverse section through the humerus just above the elbow joint.

RADIAL NERVE

Lateral

This is used for fractures of the lateral epicondyle and head of radius, for removing loose bodies from the radiohumeral joint, for the operative treatment of "tennis" elbow and in synovectomy.

- Deepen the wound in the interval between triceps posteriorly and extensor carpi radialis longus and brachioradialis anteriorly, or between extensor digitorum communis and anconeus to expose the radial head (Fig. a).

- Avoid damage to the radial nerve between brachialis and brachioradialis in the proximal part of the wound (Fig. b).

- Expose the elbow joint by detaching the common extensor origin from the lateral epicondyle. Avoid damage to the posterior interosseous nerve as it enters supinator. The posterior and/or anterior part of the joint can be exposed.

Approaches to the Elbow (continued)

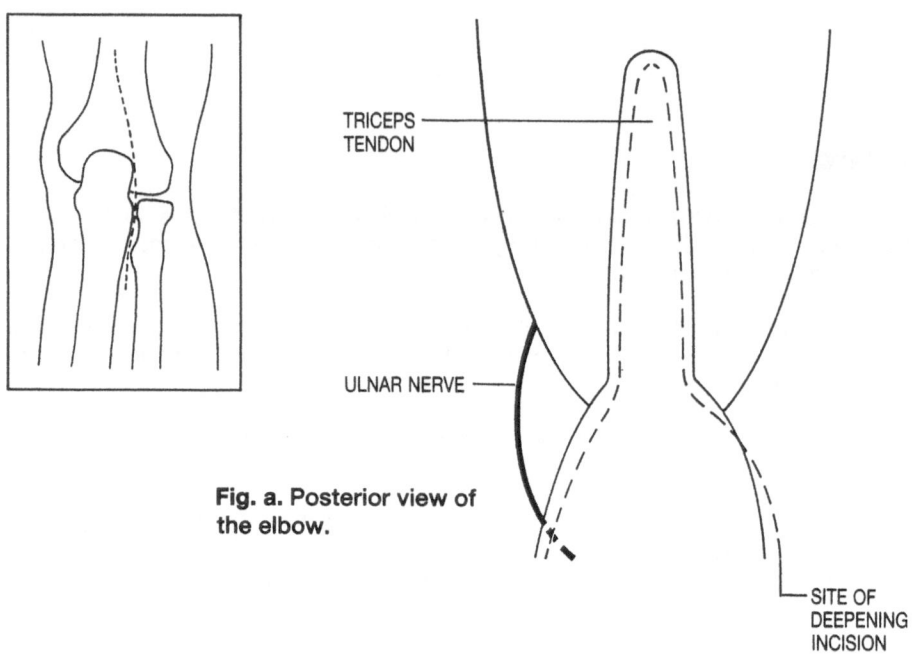

TRICEPS TENDON

ULNAR NERVE

Fig. a. Posterior view of the elbow.

SITE OF DEEPENING INCISION

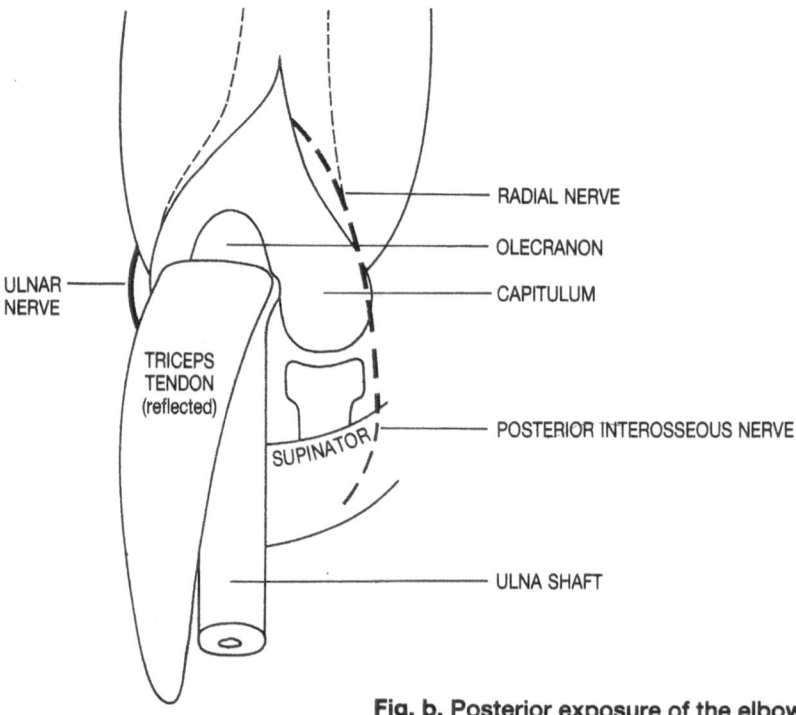

RADIAL NERVE

OLECRANON

CAPITULUM

ULNAR NERVE

TRICEPS TENDON (reflected)

SUPINATOR

POSTERIOR INTEROSSEOUS NERVE

ULNA SHAFT

Fig. b. Posterior exposure of the elbow joint.

Posterior

This can be used for elbow arthroplasty, complex distal humeral fractures, and intramedullary fixation of humeral shaft fractures.

- Identify and protect the ulnar nerve lying on the medial epicondyle (Fig. a).

- Detach the "V" shaped triceps tendon from its muscle belly leaving the base attached to the olecranon.

- Turn the triceps tendon distally, to expose the olecranon fossa and the posterior capsule (Fig. b).

- Strip the muscle fibres of triceps from the humerus. The exposure is limited proximally by the radial nerve.

- Also avoid damaging the radial nerve as it lies laterally under brachioradialis (Fig. b).

Approaches to the Elbow (continued)

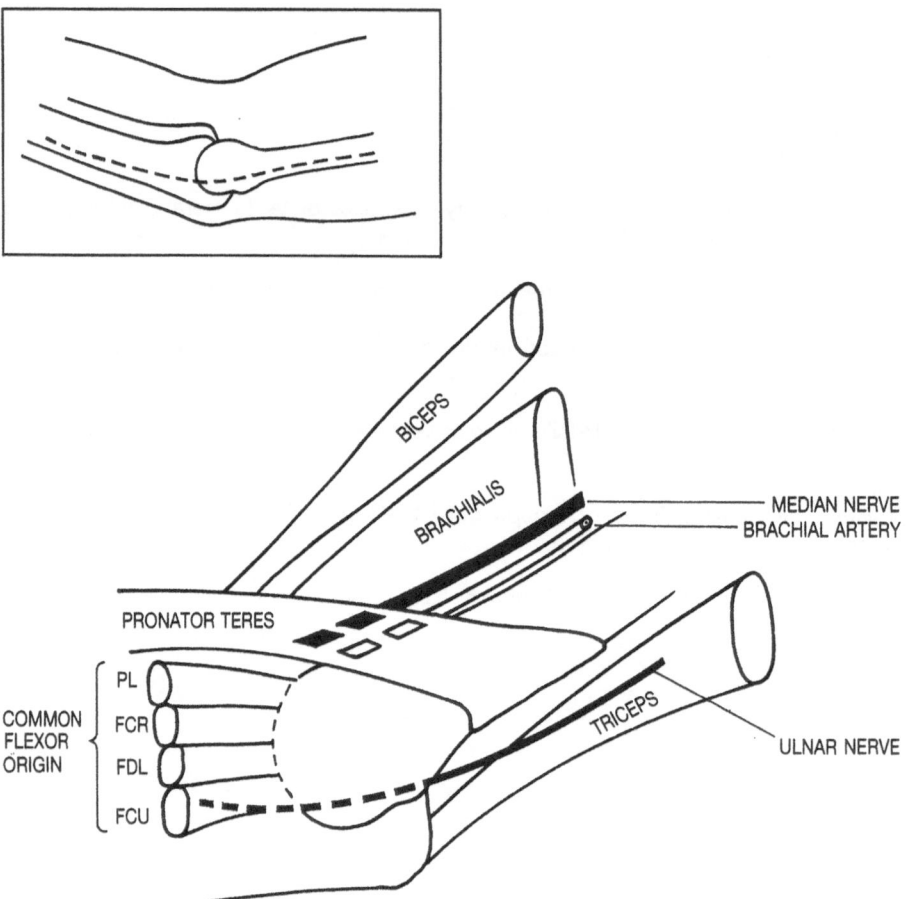

Fig. c. Medial view of the elbow.

BICEPS

BRACHIALIS

MEDIAN NERVE
BRACHIAL ARTERY

PRONATOR TERES

COMMON
FLEXOR
ORIGIN
- PL
- FCR
- FDL
- FCU

TRICEPS

ULNAR NERVE

Medial

This approach is used for releasing or transposing the ulnar nerve from the cubital tunnel, and in the treatment of "golfer's" elbow. It is also used for fractures of the medial epicondyle.

- Isolate and protect the ulnar nerve (Fig. c).

- Detach the common flexor origin from the medial epicondyle. The median nerve, the brachial artery and their branches lie deep to these muscles.

- Incise capsule and release it subperiosteally from the humerus.

Approaches to the Forearm

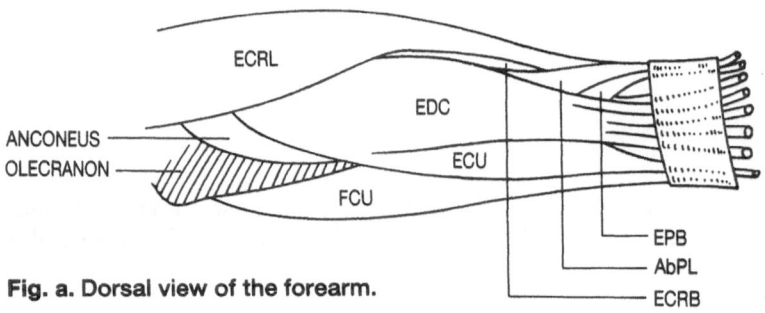

Fig. a. Dorsal view of the forearm.

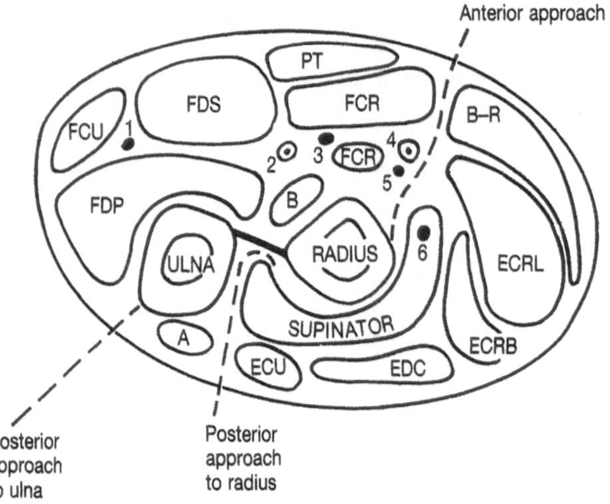

ECRL

EDC

ANCONEUS

OLECRANON

ECU

FCU

EPB

AbPL

ECRB

Anterior approach

PT

FDS

FCR

B–R

FCU 1

2 3 FCR 4

5

FDP

B

ULNA

RADIUS 6

ECRL

SUPINATOR

A

ECU

EDC

ECRB

1. Ulnar nerve
2. Ulnar artery
3. Median nerve
4. Radial artery
5. Radial nerve
6. Posterior interosseous nerve
7. Anterior interosseous nerve & artery

Posterior approach to ulna

Posterior approach to radius

(i) At level of triceps tubercle.

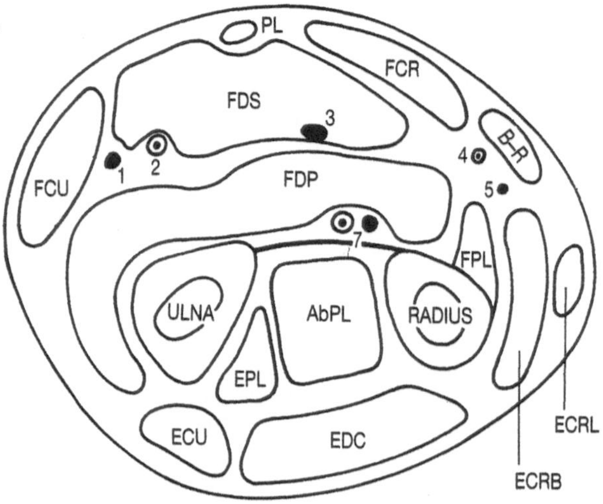

PL

FCR

FDS

3

FCU

1 2

B–R

4

5

FDP

7

FPL

ULNA

AbPL

RADIUS

EPL

ECRL

Fig. b. Transverse sections through the forearm.

ECU

EDC

ECRB

(ii) At level of mid-forearm.

Ulna

The ulna lies subcutaneously on the posterior surface of the forearm throughout its length and can be exposed direct.

- Incise longitudinally directly onto the bone.

- Expose the shaft by stripping off the flexor carpi ulnaris anteriorly and the extensor carpi ulnaris laterally (Fig. a).

Radius

In its middle and distal thirds the radius can be exposed direct through a dorsal incision, between extensor digitorum communis and extensor carpi radialis brevis. The proximal third is more difficult because of the posterior interosseous nerve. This approach should be avoided if the ulna is also to be exposed as it leaves a narrow skin bridge (Fig. b i).

Approaches to the Forearm (continued)

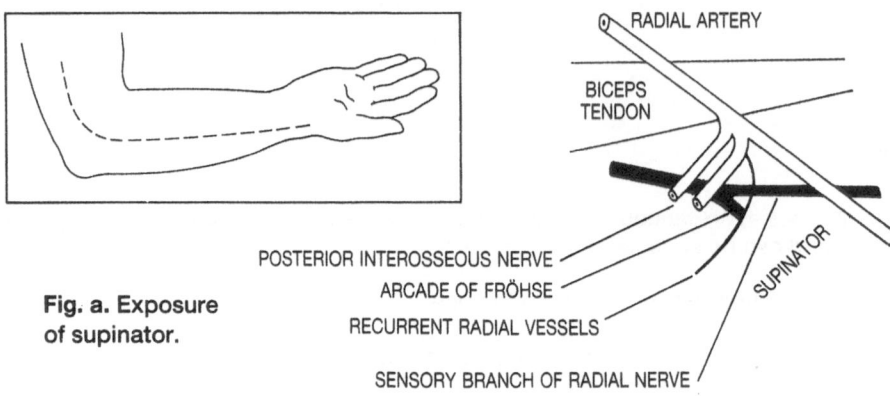

Fig. a. Exposure of supinator.

RADIAL ARTERY

BICEPS TENDON

POSTERIOR INTEROSSEOUS NERVE

ARCADE OF FRÖHSE

RECURRENT RADIAL VESSELS

SENSORY BRANCH OF RADIAL NERVE

SUPINATOR

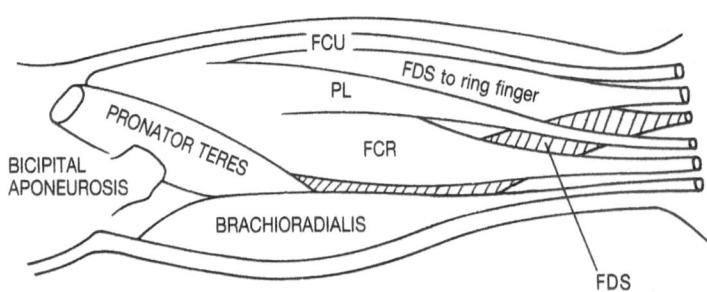

FCU

FDS to ring finger

PL

FCR

PRONATOR TERES

BICIPITAL APONEUROSIS

BRACHIORADIALIS

FDS

Fig. b. The superficial forearm flexors.

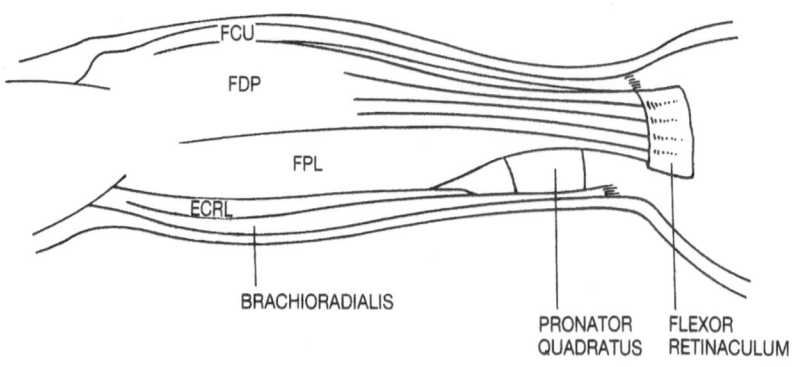

FCU

FDP

FPL

ECRL

BRACHIORADIALIS

PRONATOR QUADRATUS

FLEXOR RETINACULUM

Fig. c. The deep forearm flexors.

Anterior

All or part of this approach can be used.

Proximal

- Supinate the forearm.

- Expose the biceps tendon on its lateral side. Identify and ligate the recurrent radial vessels (Fig. a).

- Incise the bicipital bursa between the biceps tendon and the radius, and strip supinator laterally with the posterior interosseous nerve (Fig. a).

Distal

- Approach the radius between the brachioradialis and flexor carpi radialis (Fig. b ii, page 22). FCR and the muscles medial to it are innervated by the median nerve. Brachioradialis and the muscles posterior to it are innervated by the radial nerve.

- Identify the sensory branch of the radial nerve and radial artery under brachioradialis (Fig. b opposite and Fig. b ii, page 22). The nerve and artery are retracted medially with FCR.

- The flexor digitorum profundus, flexor pollicis longus, and pronator quadratus are now exposed. Strip them subperiosteally from the radius starting anterolaterally (Fig. c).

Approaches to the Wrist

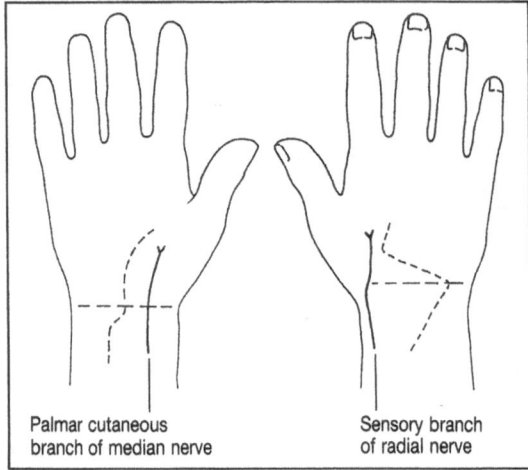

Palmar cutaneous
branch of median nerve

Sensory branch
of radial nerve

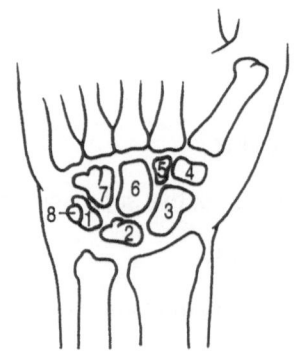

1. Triquetral	5. Trapezoid
2. Lunate	6. Capitate
3. Scaphoid	7. Hamate
4. Trapezium	8. Pisiform

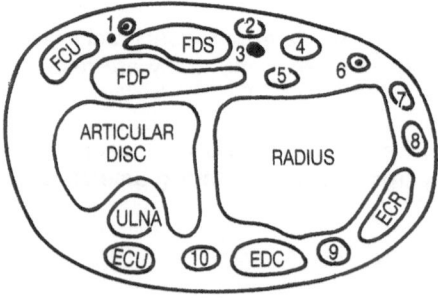

1. Ulnar nerve & artery	6. Radial artery
2. PL	7. AbPL
3. Median nerve	8. EPB
4. FCR	9. EPL
5. FPL	10. ED minimi

(i) At level of ulna styloid.

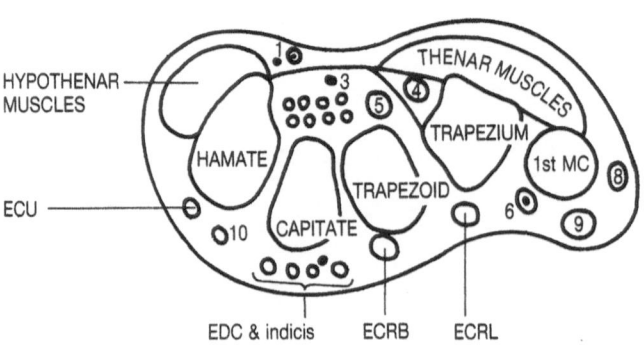

HYPOTHENAR
MUSCLES

ECU

EDC & indicis   ECRB   ECRL

Fig. a. Transverse sections through the wrist.

(ii) Through carpus.

Volar

This is most commonly performed to expose the median nerve and flexor tendons in the carpal tunnel. It is also used to reduce a dislocated lunate and in synovectomy.

- The skin incision should not encroach on the radial side of the midline to avoid damage to the palmar cutaneous branch of the median nerve.

- Incise the flexor retinaculum (transcarpal ligament) in the midline to expose the contents of the carpal tunnel (Fig. a). The median nerve is distinguished from the tendons by the vessel running within the epineurium and lies directly below palmaris longus if present.

- The superficial palmar arch crosses in the distal part of the incision (Fig. d, page 32).

- Retract the median nerve, palmaris longus and flexor pollicis longus radially, and the tendons of flexor digitorum sublimis and flexor digitorum profundus ulnarwards to expose the capsule and the carpus.

- The lunate lies in the midline proximal to the capitate (Fig. a).

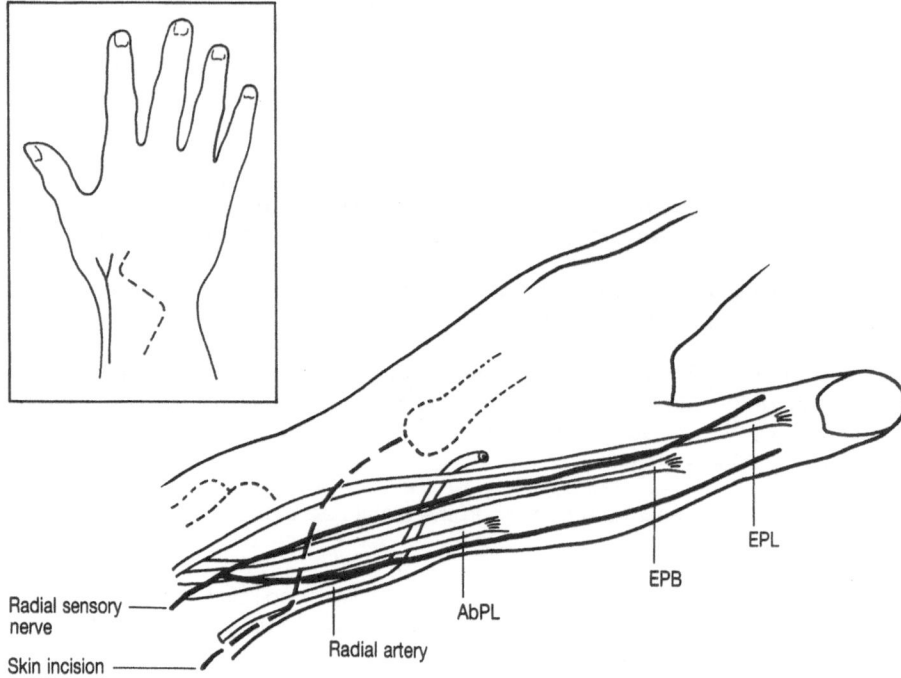

Radial sensory nerve

Skin incision

Radial artery

AbPL

EPB

EPL

Fig. a. Lateral view of the wrist and dorsum of the thumb.

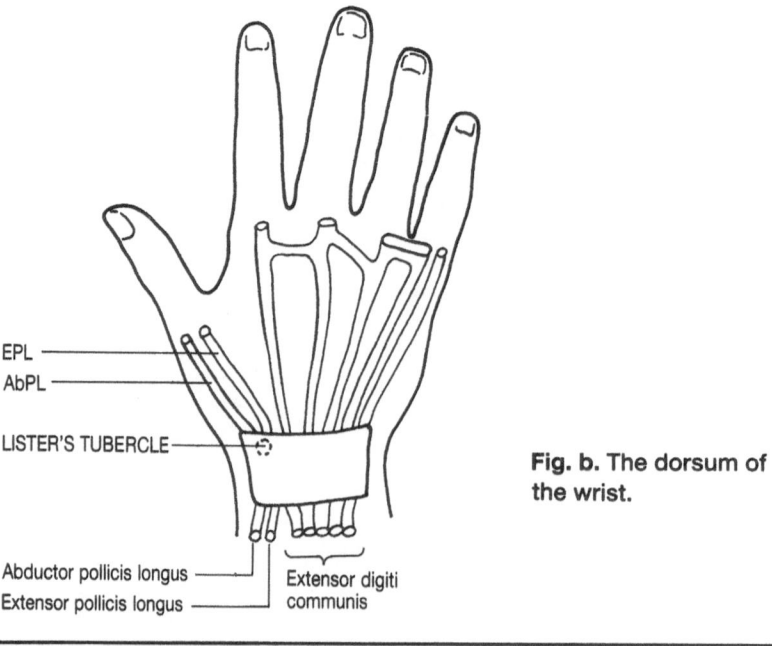

EPL

AbPL

LISTER'S TUBERCLE

Fig. b. The dorsum of the wrist.

Abductor pollicis longus

Extensor pollicis longus

Extensor digiti communis

Lateral

This is useful for exposing the scaphoid in cases of nonunion, or in exposing the trapezium.

- Deepen the wound taking care not to damage the sensory branches of the radial nerve (Fig. a).

- Retract the nerve, extensor pollicis brevis, the thumb abductors, and the radial artery volarly. Retract the extensor pollicis longus dorsally. The tubercle of the scaphoid is now exposed.

- Divide the radial collateral ligament and capsule longitudinally to expose the joint.

Dorsal

This approach to the wrist is used in arthrodesis or arthroplasty of the wrist, and in exposure of the extensor tendons.

- Centre the incisions on Lister's tubercle (Fig. b).

- Deepen the wound through the extensor retinaculum dividing it along its ulna attachment taking care not to damage extensor pollicis longus as it curves round the tubercle.

- Retract the finger extensors ulnarwards.

- Incise the capsule transversely.

Approaches to the Hand

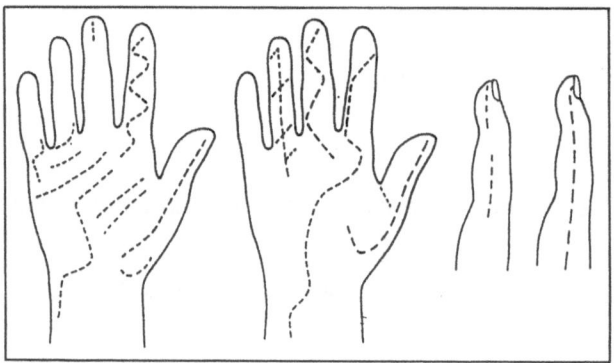

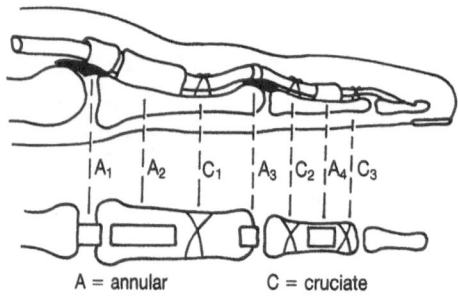

A = annular   C = cruciate

Fig. a. The flexor tendon pulley system.

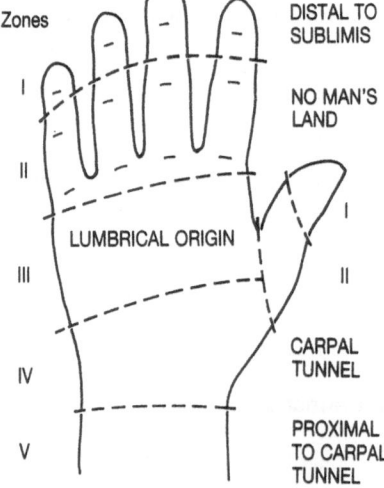

Zones

I

II

LUMBRICAL ORIGIN

III

IV

V

DISTAL TO SUBLIMIS

NO MAN'S LAND

I

II

CARPAL TUNNEL

PROXIMAL TO CARPAL TUNNEL

Fig. b. Zones for the flexor tendons.

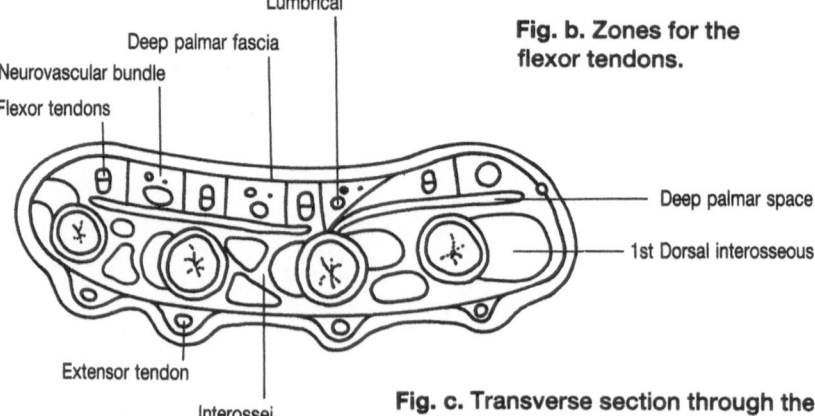

Lumbrical

Deep palmar fascia

Neurovascular bundle

Flexor tendons

Deep palmar space

1st Dorsal interosseous

Extensor tendon

Interossei

Fig. c. Transverse section through the metacarpals.

The standard hand incisions are shown.

Exposure of Palm and Digit

The incision depends on which parts of the palm and digit need to be exposed (see inset). All or part of each incision illustrated may be used.

- In flexor tendon injuries it is important to preserve the A2 and A4 pulleys (Fig. a opposite and Fig. d, page 32) to prevent bowstringing during flexion. If this occurs the increased moment arm leads to reduced power. The palmar aponeurosis and the flexor retinaculum also act as pulleys. As a result, when the proximal part of the tendon is retracted from the site of the wound, it is better to make multiple small incisions to find it rather than a long digital and palmar wound incising the palmar fascia and flexor retinaculum.

- The site of flexor tendon injury is described by zones (Fig. b). Those in zone II, which begins at the distal palmar skin crease and finishes at the insertion of sublimis, should be repaired by experts. Zone II in the thumb begins at the proximal thumb skin crease and ends at the A2 pulley.

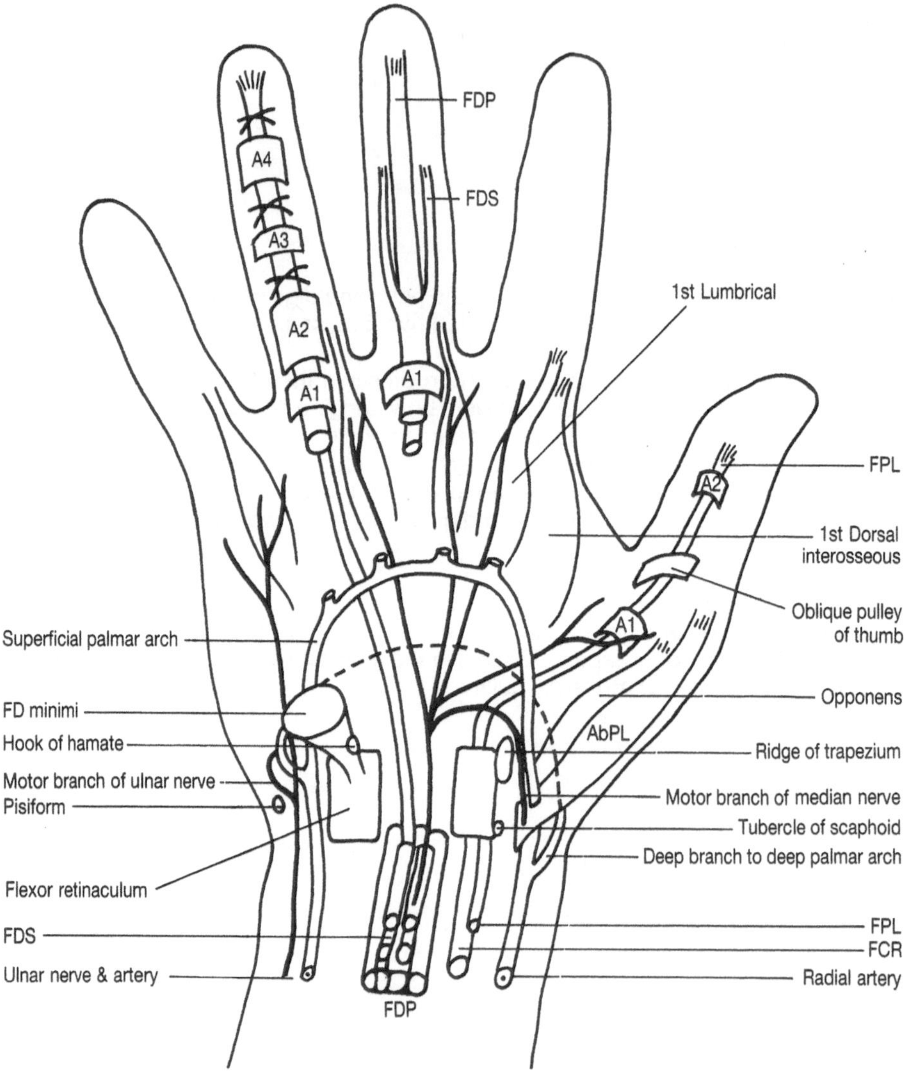

FDP

A4

A3

A2

A1

A1

1st Lumbrical

FPL

A2

1st Dorsal
interosseous

Oblique pulley
of thumb

A1

Superficial palmar arch

Opponens

FD minimi

AbPL

Hook of hamate

Ridge of trapezium

Motor branch of ulnar nerve

Pisiform

Motor branch of median nerve

Tubercle of scaphoid

Deep branch to deep palmar arch

Flexor retinaculum

FDS

FPL

FCR

Ulnar nerve & artery

Radial artery

FDP

Fig. d. Structures of the palmar surface of the hand.

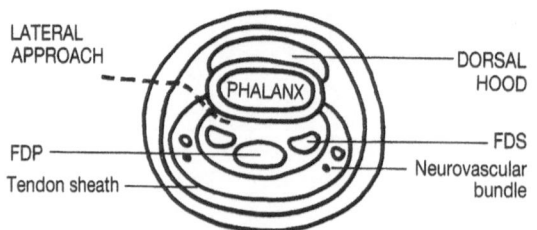

LATERAL
APPROACH

DORSAL
HOOD

PHALANX

FDS

FDP

Tendon sheath

Neurovascular
bundle

**Fig. e. Transverse section
through digit.**

- In Dupuytren's disease the digital nerves are often surrounded by thickened palmar fascia. Note that the radial digital nerve to the index and little fingers passes in front of the metacarpophalangeal joint (Fig. c, page 30 and Fig. d opposite).

- In trigger finger the A1 pulley is divided.

- The flexor sheath can be approached by a lateral incision (Fig. e). This is useful for some benign tumours and also in tenolysis of the tendons or to expose the phalanges or joints.

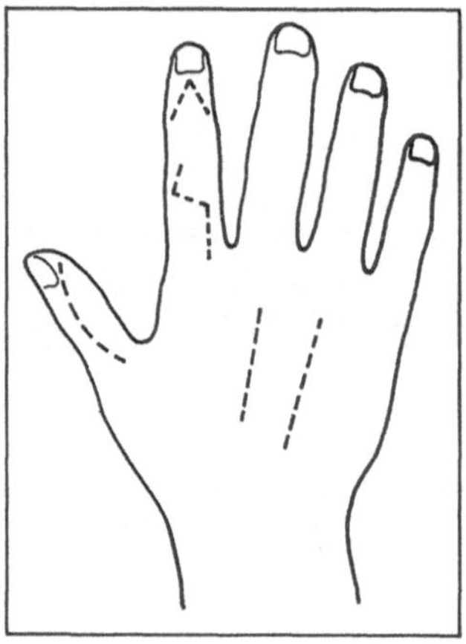

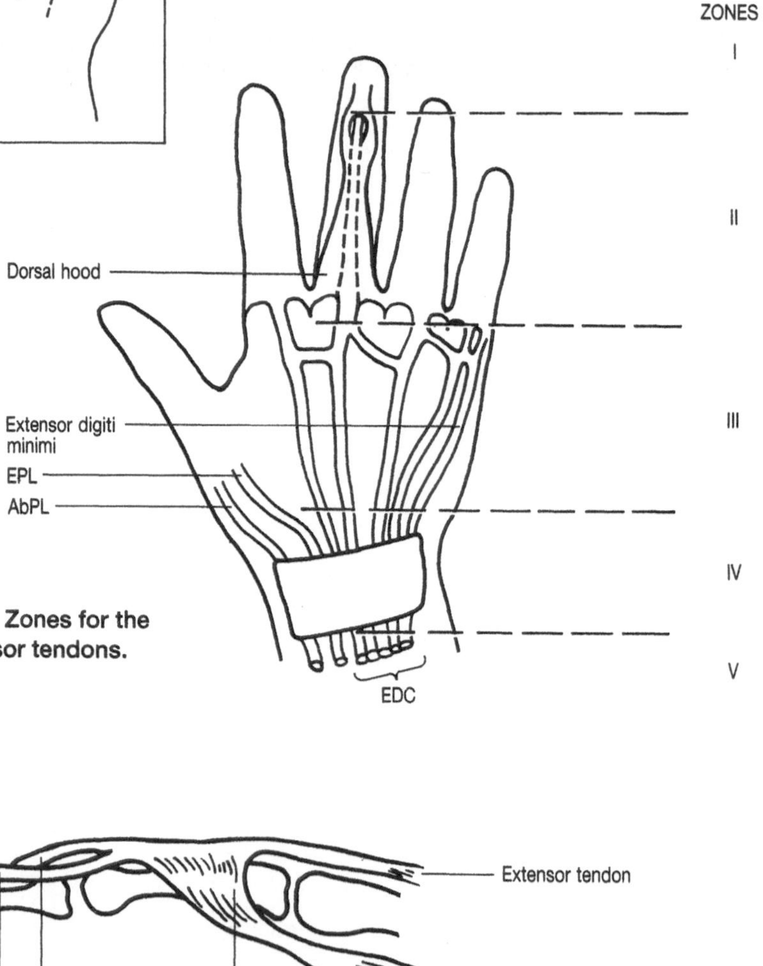

Dorsal hood

Extensor digiti minimi

EPL

AbPL

Fig. a. Zones for the extensor tendons.

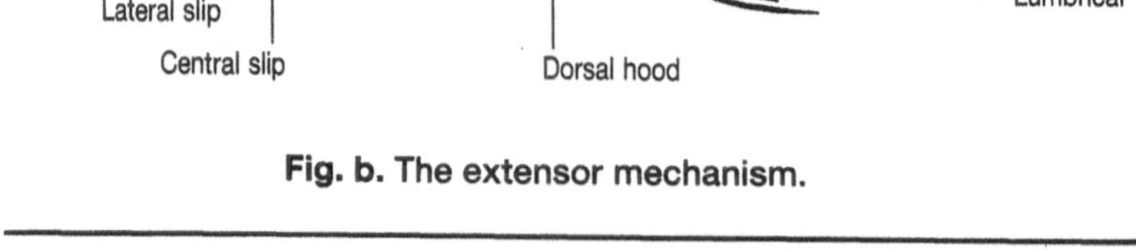

EDC

ZONES

I

II

III

IV

V

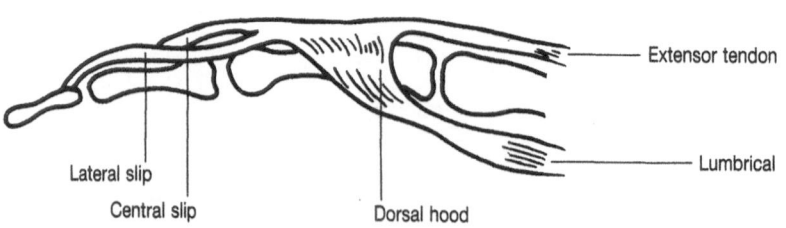

Lateral slip

Central slip

Dorsal hood

Extensor tendon

Lumbrical

Fig. b. The extensor mechanism.

Dorsum of the Hand

These are described by zones (Fig. a) which relate to the middle finger. The extensor mechanism is complex (Fig. b). The long extensor tendon extends the metacarpophalangeal (MCP) joint, the lumbrical stops hyperextension of the MCP joint and extends the interphalangeal joints.

Zone I lies distal to the insertion of the central slip into the middle phalanx, zone II begins just proximal to the MCP joints and includes the dorsal hood, zone III lies on the dorsum of the hand, zone IV is under the extensor retinaculum of the wrist, and zone V lies proximal to this.

- Repairs in zone I are usually unnecessary.

- Repairs in zone II are difficult. Beware of damage to the central slip at the proximal interphalangeal joint as failure to repair this leads to a Boutonnière deformity.

II. Lower Limb

Approaches to the Hip

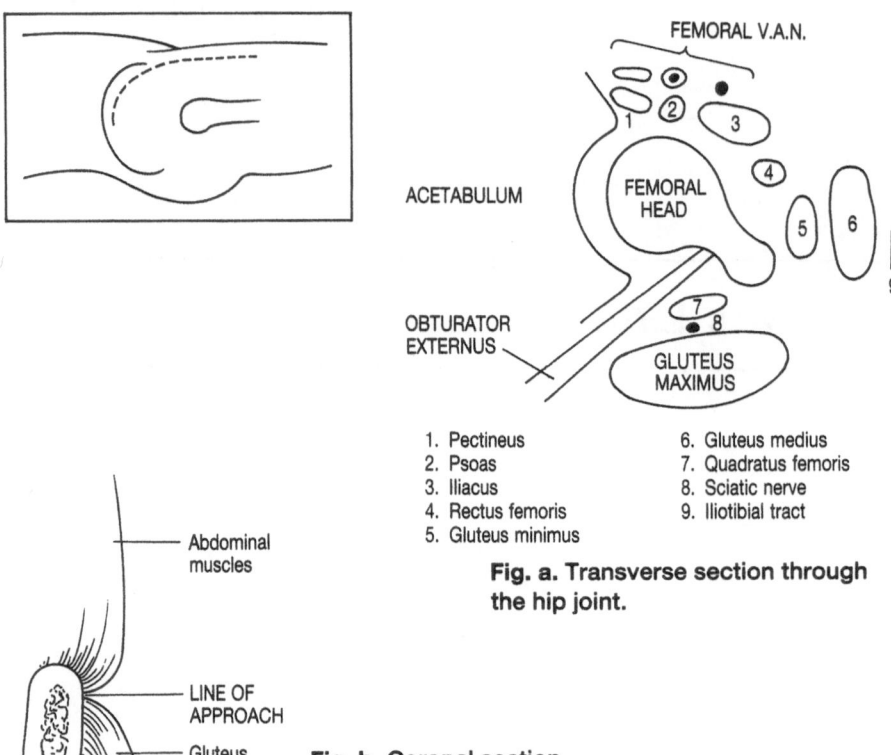

FEMORAL V.A.N.

ACETABULUM

FEMORAL HEAD

OBTURATOR EXTERNUS

GLUTEUS MAXIMUS

1. Pectineus
2. Psoas
3. Iliacus
4. Rectus femoris
5. Gluteus minimus
6. Gluteus medius
7. Quadratus femoris
8. Sciatic nerve
9. Iliotibial tract

Fig. a. Transverse section through the hip joint.

Abdominal muscles

LINE OF APPROACH

Gluteus medius

Fig. b. Coronal section of iliac wing.

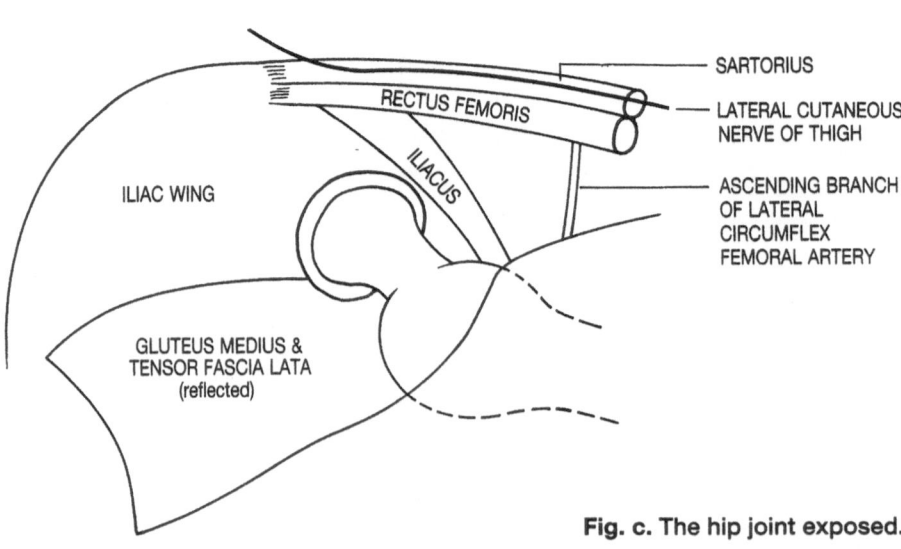

SARTORIUS

RECTUS FEMORIS

LATERAL CUTANEOUS NERVE OF THIGH

ILIACUS

ASCENDING BRANCH OF LATERAL CIRCUMFLEX FEMORAL ARTERY

ILIAC WING

GLUTEUS MEDIUS & TENSOR FASCIA LATA (reflected)

Fig. c. The hip joint exposed.

There are many described approaches to the hip joint; the most popular are the posterior and the lateral. These are most commonly used for arthroplasty of the joint.

Anterior (Iliofemoral)

- Centre the incision on the anterior superior iliac spine.

- Detach the gluteus medius and tensor fascia lata from the iliac crest and then subperiosteally from the iliac wing down to the acetabulum.

- Retract rectus femoris and sartorius medially with the lateral cutaneous nerve of the thigh. (See Fig. c.)

- Ligate and divide the ascending branch of the lateral circumflex femoral artery as it lies in the distal part of the wound.

- Expose the capsule of the hip joint by reflecting the gluteus medius and tensor fascia lata posteriorly.

- Incise the capsule and dislocate the hip joint by externally rotating and adducting the leg.

The iliac crest part of the incision is also used to expose the iliac crest for obtaining donor bone (Fig. b). In open reduction for CDH, rectus femoris is divided and reflected inferiorly.

Approaches to the Hip (continued)

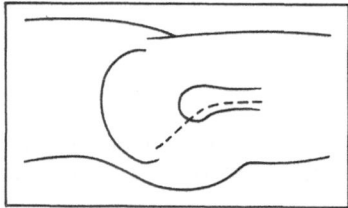

1. Retract anterior border of gluteus medius
2. Detach insertion of gluteus medius (& minimus)
3. Perform a trochanteric osteotomy (see Fig. b)
4. Split gluteus medius & vastus lateralis in line of fibres

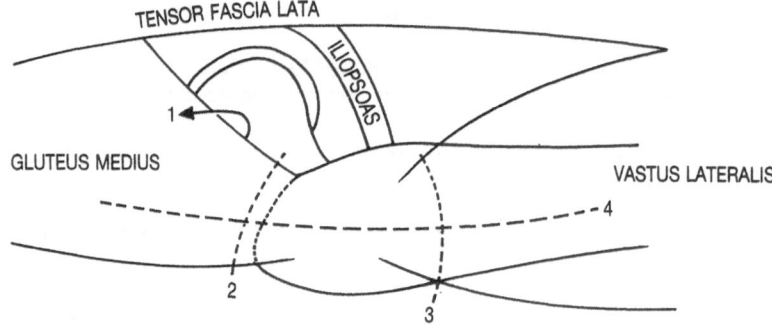

Fig. a. Lateral approaches to the hip joint.

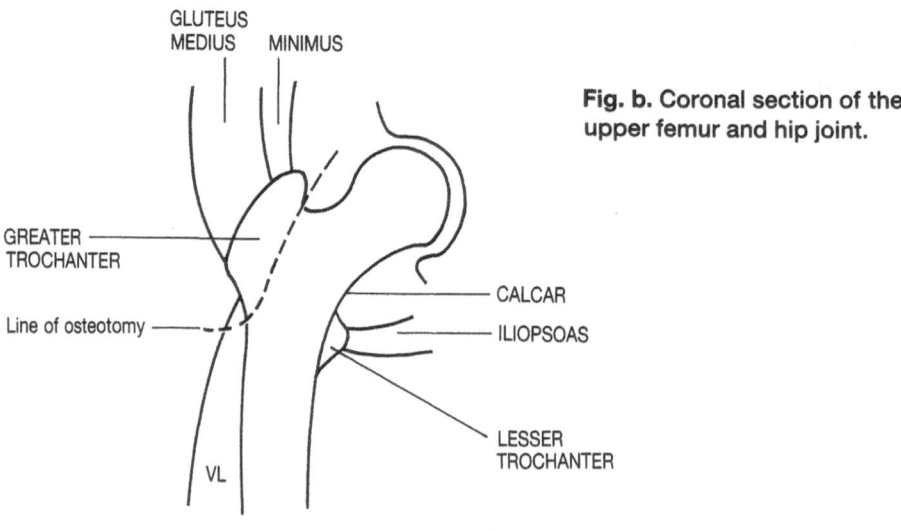

Fig. b. Coronal section of the upper femur and hip joint.

Lateral

The only true lateral approach to the hip is via detachment of the greater trochanter. The other three approaches described are strictly speaking anterolateral approaches. However they only vary in how gluteus medius is reflected to expose the hip joint.

- Centre the incision on the tip of the greater trochanter.

- Divide the gluteal fascia and iliotibial tract to expose gluteus medius and vastus lateralis.

- Expose the hip joint by (Fig. a):

  either 1. retracting the anterior border of gluteus medius supero-posteriorly.

  or   2. dividing gluteus medius and minimus at their tendinous insertion into the greater trochanter and retracting them superiorly.

  or   3. performing a trochanteric osteotomy and retracting the greater trochanter superiorly (Fig. b).

  or   4. performing a muscle-splitting incision into gluteus medius and vastus lateralis and retracting them anteriorly.

- Incise the capsule and dislocate the hip joint by externally rotating and adducting the leg.

The upper part of the fourth approach, separating the gluteus medius in the line of its fibres, allows access to the piriform fossa, which is just posteromedial to the tip of the greater trochanter. This is the entry point for a straight-stemmed femoral prosthesis or intramedullary nail which should be aimed forwards as the femur has an anterior bow.

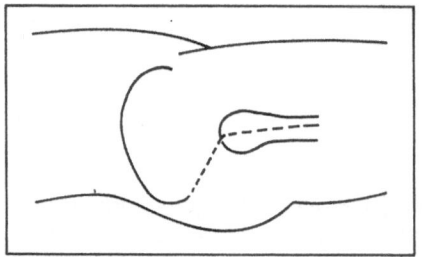

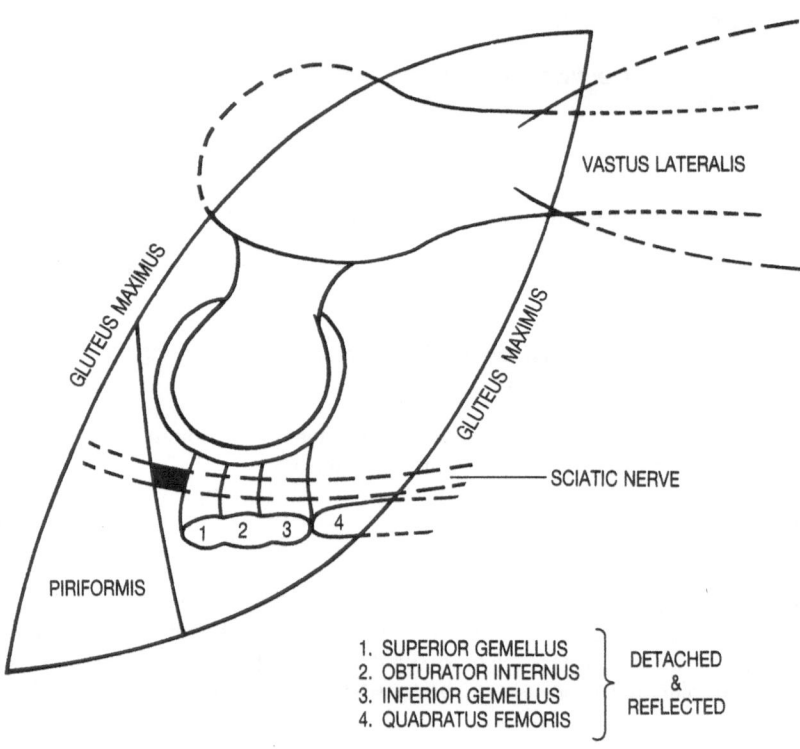

GLUTEUS MAXIMUS

GLUTEUS MAXIMUS

VASTUS LATERALIS

SCIATIC NERVE

PIRIFORMIS

1. SUPERIOR GEMELLUS
2. OBTURATOR INTERNUS
3. INFERIOR GEMELLUS
4. QUADRATUS FEMORIS

} DETACHED & REFLECTED

Fig. a. Posterior exposure of the hip joint.

Posterior

This is the most popular approach for performing an hemiarthroplasty for subcapital fractures of the neck of the femur. Place the patient in the lateral position. Centre the incision on the tip of the greater trochanter.

- Split the gluteus maximus in the line of its fibres.

- Identify the sciatic nerve deep to the gluteus maximus as it emerges from under piriformis. Protect it by detaching the short rotator muscles from the femur and turning them posteriorly (Fig. a).

- Incise the capsule and dislocate the hip joint by internally rotating, flexing, and adducting the leg.

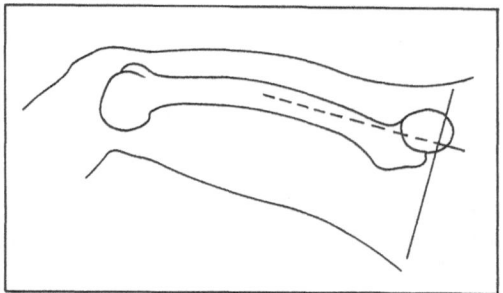

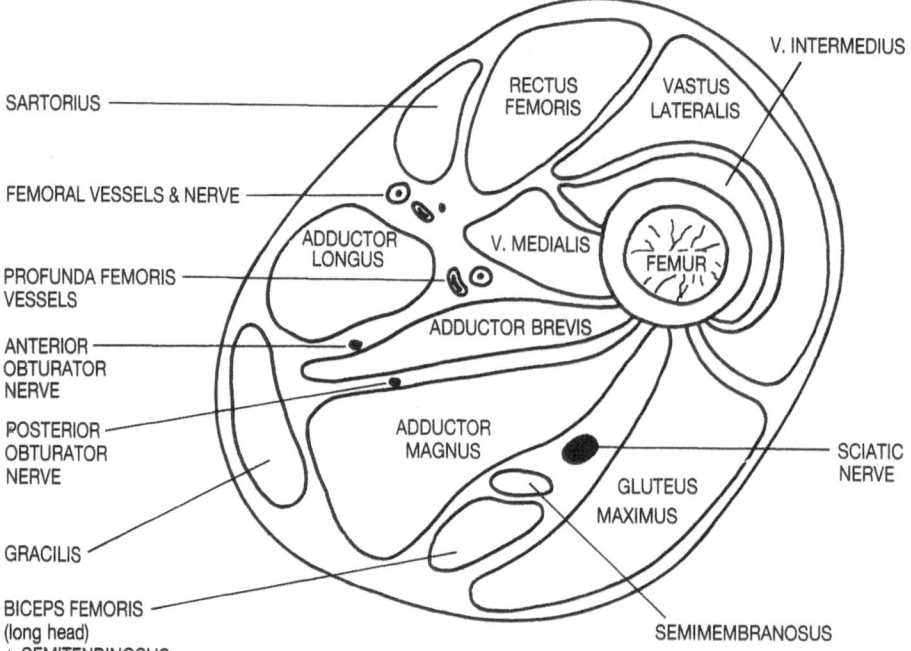

SARTORIUS

RECTUS FEMORIS

VASTUS LATERALIS

V. INTERMEDIUS

FEMORAL VESSELS & NERVE

V. MEDIALIS

FEMUR

ADDUCTOR LONGUS

PROFUNDA FEMORIS VESSELS

ADDUCTOR BREVIS

ANTERIOR OBTURATOR NERVE

POSTERIOR OBTURATOR NERVE

ADDUCTOR MAGNUS

SCIATIC NERVE

GLUTEUS MAXIMUS

GRACILIS

BICEPS FEMORIS (long head) + SEMITENDINOSUS

SEMIMEMBRANOSUS

Fig. a. Transverse section through the upper femur.

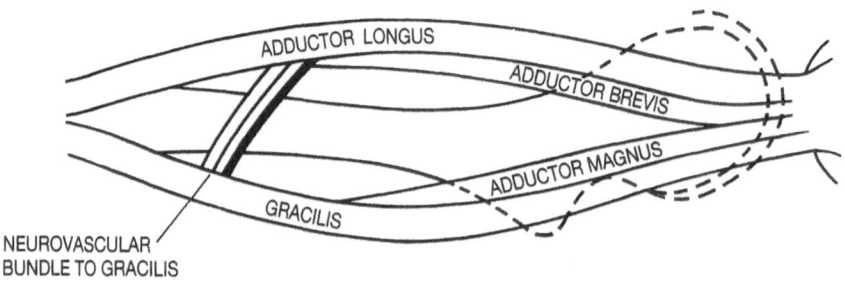

ADDUCTOR LONGUS

ADDUCTOR BREVIS

ADDUCTOR MAGNUS

GRACILIS

NEUROVASCULAR BUNDLE TO GRACILIS

Fig. b. Medial exposure of the hip joint.

Medial

This is an unusual approach designed for the reduction of the congenitally dislocated hip. The initial part is used for adductor tenotomy and obturator neurectomy in cerebral palsy.

- Flex, abduct, and externally rotate the hip. This halves the amount of soft tissue between the skin and the hip.

- Begin the skin incision 2.5 cm distal to the pubic tubercle and descend longitudinally between gracilis and adductor longus.

- Deepen the wound between adductor longus plus adductor brevis and gracilis plus adductor magnus (Fig. a).

- Avoid damage to the posterior branch of the obturator nerve as it lies on adductor magnus.

- Avoid damage to the neurovascular supply to gracilis in the distal part of the incision (Fig. b).

- Incise the capsule to expose the femoral head in the bed of the wound.

Approaches to the Proximal Femur

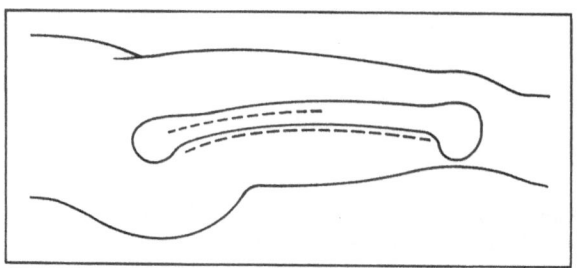

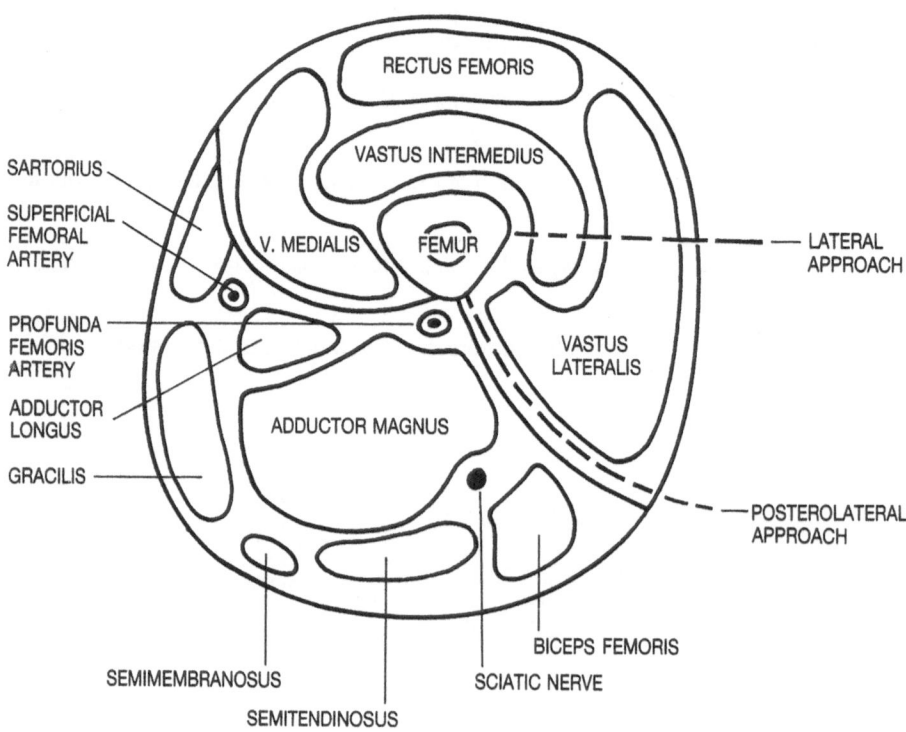

Fig. a. Transverse section through the middle of the thigh.

Approaches to the Proximal Femur

These approaches are most commonly used internally to fix fractures of the femur. They are also used for an upper femoral osteotomy.

The incision extends distally from the tip of the greater trochanter to the proximal part of the shaft of the femur. A slightly more posterior incision allows exposure of the shaft which avoids dividing muscle. The whole shaft can be exposed this way.

Lateral

- Divide the fascia lata immediately posterior to the fibres of tensor fascia lata.

- Split the vastus lateralis in the line of its fibres down to bone. (Fig. a opposite and Fig. a, page 44).

Posterolateral

- After incision of the fascia lata identify the lateral intermuscular septum and trace it posteriorly to the linea aspera.

- Separate the lateral intermuscular septum from the vastus lateralis which is then retracted anteriorly and stripped from the surface of the bone.

Approaches to the Distal Femur

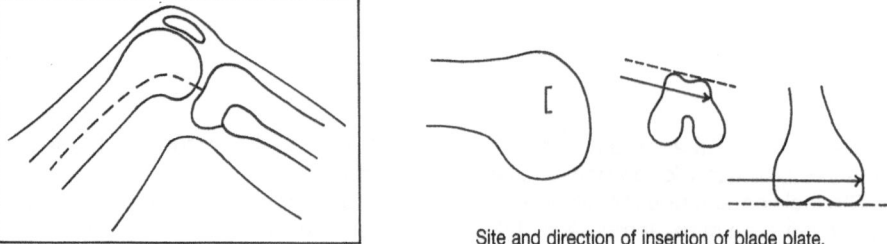

Site and direction of insertion of blade plate.

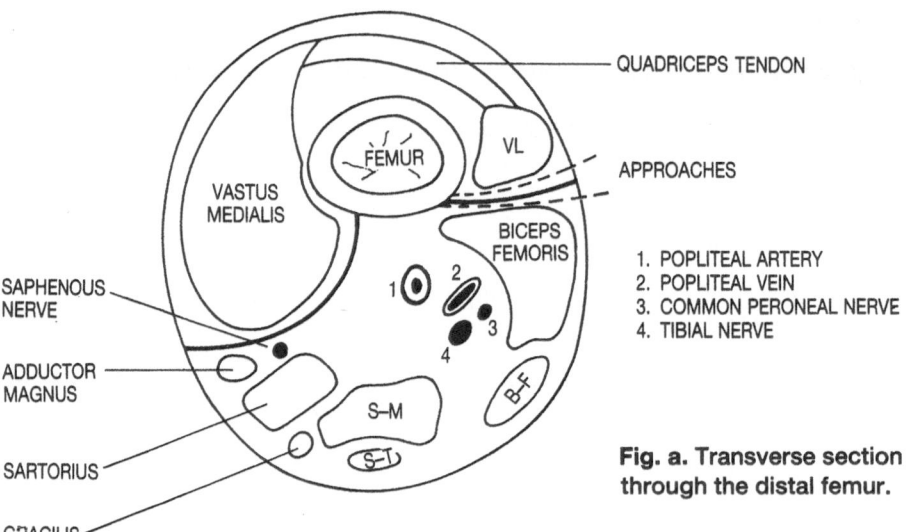

QUADRICEPS TENDON

VL

FEMUR

VASTUS MEDIALIS

APPROACHES

BICEPS FEMORIS

SAPHENOUS NERVE

1. POPLITEAL ARTERY
2. POPLITEAL VEIN
3. COMMON PERONEAL NERVE
4. TIBIAL NERVE

ADDUCTOR MAGNUS

B-F

SARTORIUS

S–M

S-T

GRACILIS

Fig. a. Transverse section through the distal femur.

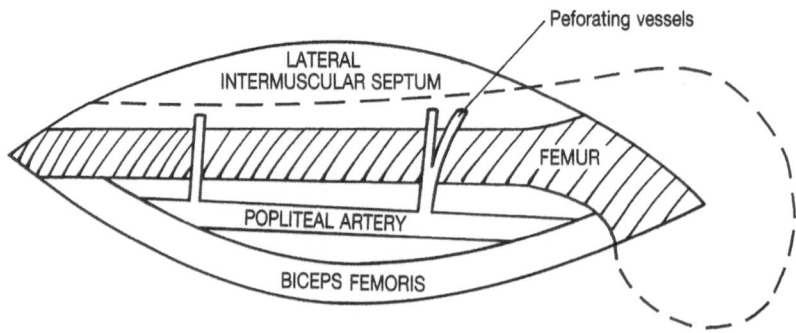

Peforating vessels

LATERAL INTERMUSCULAR SEPTUM

FEMUR

POPLITEAL ARTERY

BICEPS FEMORIS

Fig. b. Lateral exposure of the distal femur.

Approaches to the Distal Femur

The distal femur may be exposed either medially or laterally. The lateral exposure is used for blade plating supracondylar fractures. The inset shows the site of entry and direction for insertion of the blade. Note that the lateral condyle is more prominent, and that the femoral shaft inserts into the anterior part of the condyles.

Either or both approaches may be used for complex condylar fractures. For these exposures the knee should be slightly flexed to allow the popliteal vessels to fall backwards.

Lateral

To reach the anterolateral part of the femur the approach lies in front of the intermuscular septum. To reach the posterior part of the femur the approach lies behind the intermuscular septum (Fig. a).

Anterolateral Surface

● Sweep the vastus lateralis of the intermuscular septum.

● Identify and ligate the perforating vessels from the popliteal artery as they emerge close to the femur.

Posterior Surface

● Divide the deep fascia behind the iliotibial tract and separate the biceps femoris from the intermuscular septum.

● Identify and ligate the perforating vessels from the popliteal artery (Fig. b).

● Retract the popliteal vessels posteriorly and keep to bone.

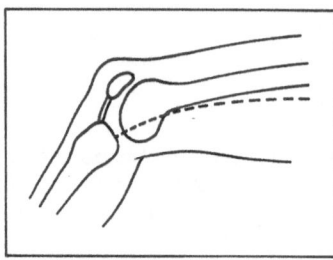

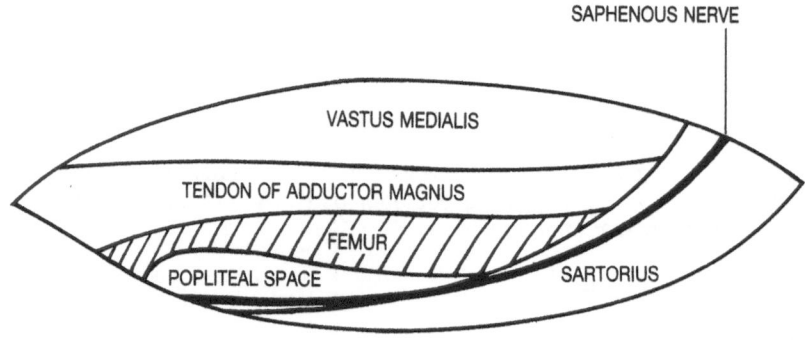

Fig. c. Medial exposure of the distal femur.

Medial

The medial, as opposed to anteromedial, exposure is preferred as the latter involves separating rectus femoris from the vastus medialis and dividing the vastus intermedius.

The incision is based on the adductor tubercle and as such should avoid the saphenous vein which runs more posteriorly.

- The synovium of the knee joint lies in the distal part of the incision deep to sartorius and anterior to the adductor tubercle, therefore divide the fascia on the anterior border of sartorius carefully. Sartorius then falls posteriorly.

- The saphenous nerve then lies on sartorius deep to the adductor magnus tendon (Fig. c).

- Get to bone by blunt dissection and retract the popliteal vessels posteriorly.

Approaches to the Knee

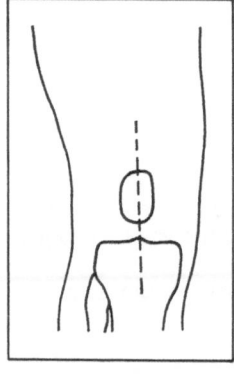

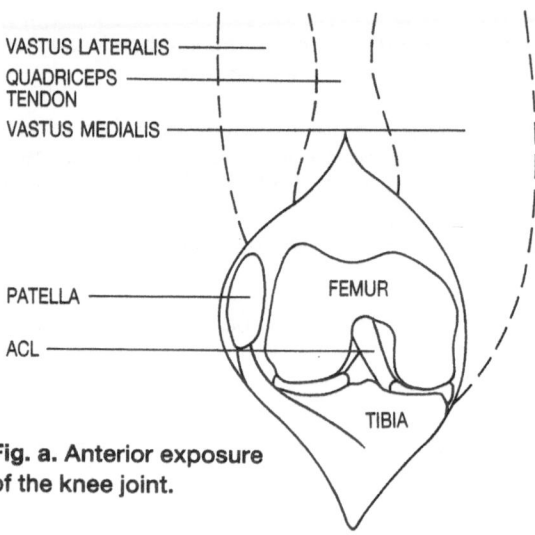

VASTUS LATERALIS

QUADRICEPS TENDON

VASTUS MEDIALIS

PATELLA

ACL

FEMUR

TIBIA

Fig. a. Anterior exposure of the knee joint.

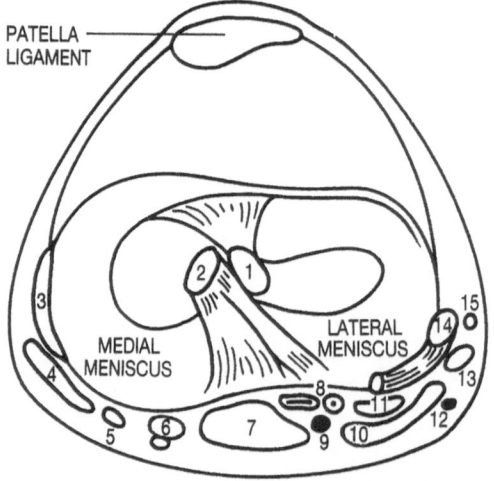

PATELLA LIGAMENT

MEDIAL MENISCUS

LATERAL MENISCUS

1. Anterior cruciate
2. Posterior cruciate
3. Medial collateral ligament
4. Sartorius
5. Gracilis
6. Semimembranosus (with semitendinosus)
7. Medial gastrocnemius
8. Popliteal vessels
9. Tibial nerve
10. Lateral gastrocnemius
11. Plantaris
12. Common peroneal nerve
13. Biceps femoris
14. Popliteus tendon
15. Lateral collateral ligament

Fig. b. Transverse section through the knee.

Anterior

This approach allows access to all but the posterior compartment of the joint. It is mainly used for knee replacement, since many intra-articular procedures are carried out through the arthroscope.

The incision runs in the true midline over the patella to the tibial tubercle.

- Separate the quadriceps tendon from the vastus medialis and continue the incision distally along the medial border of the patella and through the patella retinaculum and capsule alongside the patella ligament.

- Retract and evert the patella laterally and flex the knee joint (Fig. a).

- All the important structures lie behind the posterior capsule (Fig. b).

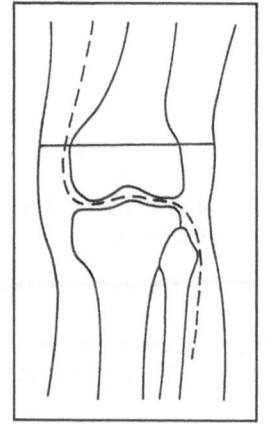

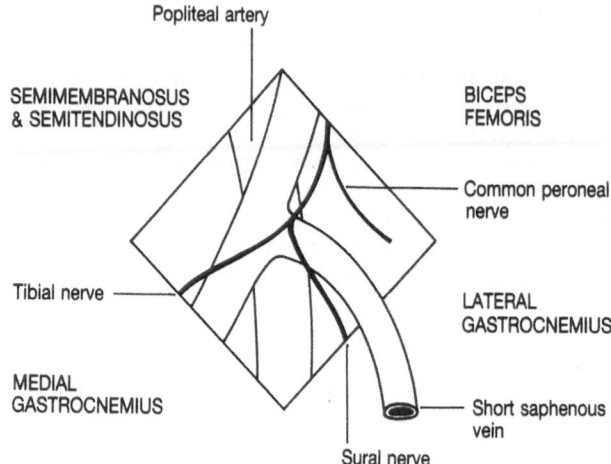

Fig. a. The popliteal fossa.

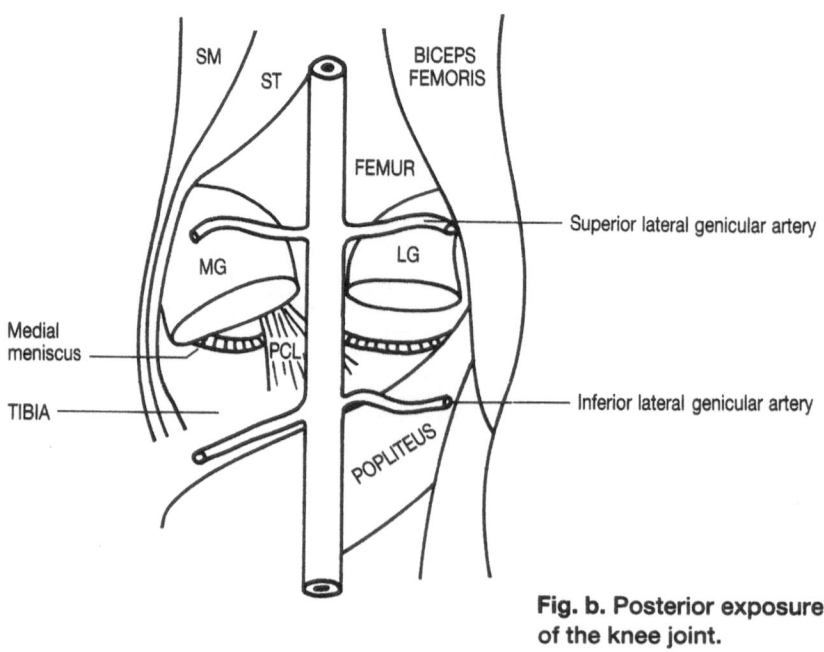

Fig. b. Posterior exposure
of the knee joint.

Posterior

This approach encounters structures that if damaged can lead to serious disability. It is used to gain access to the popliteal fossa and the posterior aspect of the knee joint. The patient lies prone.

- The flexure crease of the knee lies proximal to the knee joint. The incision is "S" shaped with the proximal limb on semitendinosus, the transverse limb over the joint line which lies distal to the flexure crease, and the distal limb over the lateral gastrocnemius.

- Locate the sural nerve between the two heads of gastrocnemius and trace it proximally to the tibial nerve and then the common peroneal nerve (Fig. a).

- Retract the nerves and expose the popliteal vein and artery. Identify the superior medial and lateral genicular vessels. Retract the vessels laterally to expose the posterior capsule (Fig. b).

- Retract semitendinosus medially and expose the attachment of the medial head of gastrocnemius and the posterior capsule.

- Incise the capsule and retract it with the attached medial head of gastrocnemius laterally to protect the nerves and vessels and enter the posteromedial part of the joint.

- Approach the posterolateral part of the joint between biceps femoris and the lateral head of gastrocnemius.

Approach to the Tibial Plateau

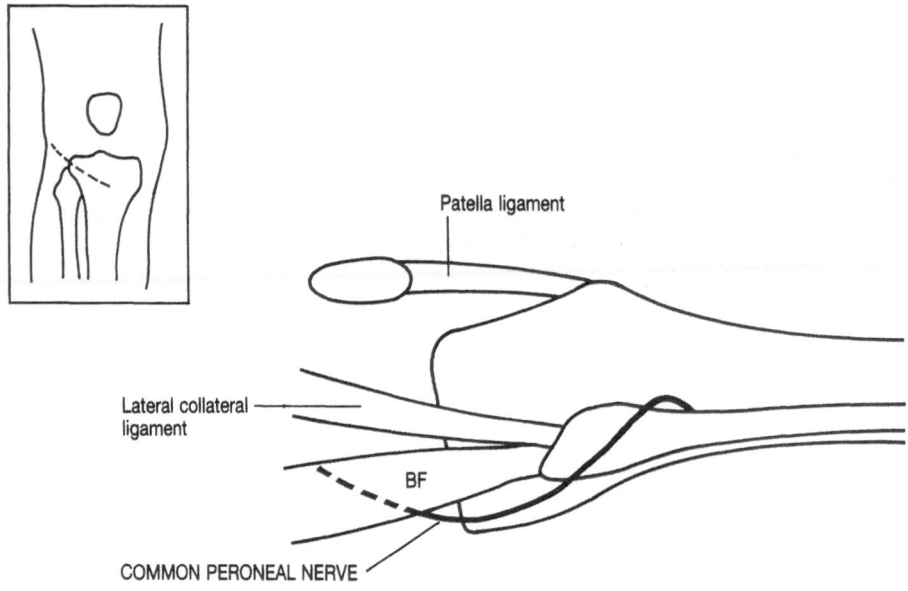

Patella ligament

Lateral collateral ligament

BF

COMMON PERONEAL NERVE

Fig. a. Lateral view of the upper tibia.

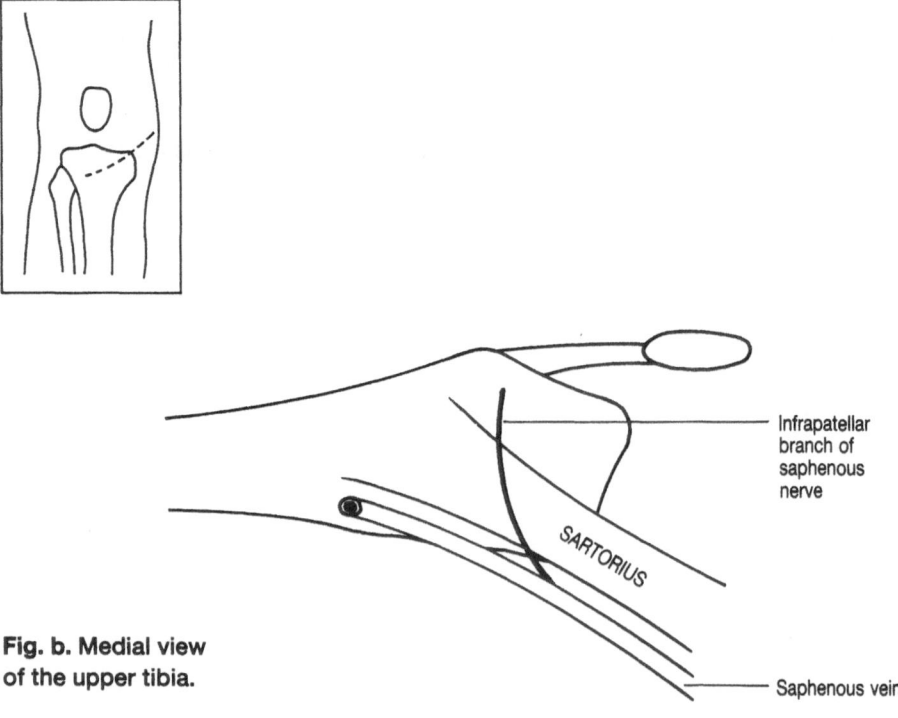

Infrapatellar branch of saphenous nerve

SARTORIUS

Fig. b. Medial view of the upper tibia.

Saphenous vein

Approach to the Tibial Plateau

This is used mainly for upper tibial osteotomy and fixing tibial plateau fractures.

A horizontal or slightly oblique incision gives satisfactory access but should not cross the midline if a longitudinal incision for a future joint arthroplasty is contemplated.

- The common peroneal nerve emerges from the medial aspect of the biceps tendon and runs laterally around the neck of the fibula deep to peroneus longus (Fig. a). It is at risk in more distal exposures.

- Identify the tibiofemoral joint by flexing the knee to 90°.

- On the medial side (Fig. b) the infrapatellar branch of the saphenous nerve may be damaged if the incision is too proximal.

- The tibial plateau is subcutaneous and is exposed on incising the skin.

Approaches to the Tibial Shaft

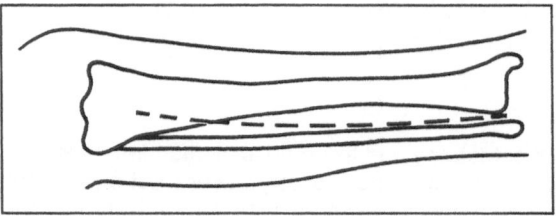

1. Posterior tibial artery
2. Peroneal artery
3. Superficial peroneal nerve
4. Deep peroneal nerve
5. Posterior tibial nerve
6. Flexor digitorum longus
7. Popliteus
8. Plantaris
9. Sural nerve
10. Anterior tibial artery

Fig. a. Transverse section of the upper calf.

Anterior

This is used for plating fractures or biopsying tumours and anterior fasciotomy for compartment syndrome.

- The incision is placed lateral to the tibial crest over the tibialis anterior muscle. The anteromedial surface is subcutaneous.

- Expose the lateral surface by stripping tibialis anterior from the bone (Fig. a, opposite and Fig. b, page 60).

Approaches to the Tibial Shaft (continued)

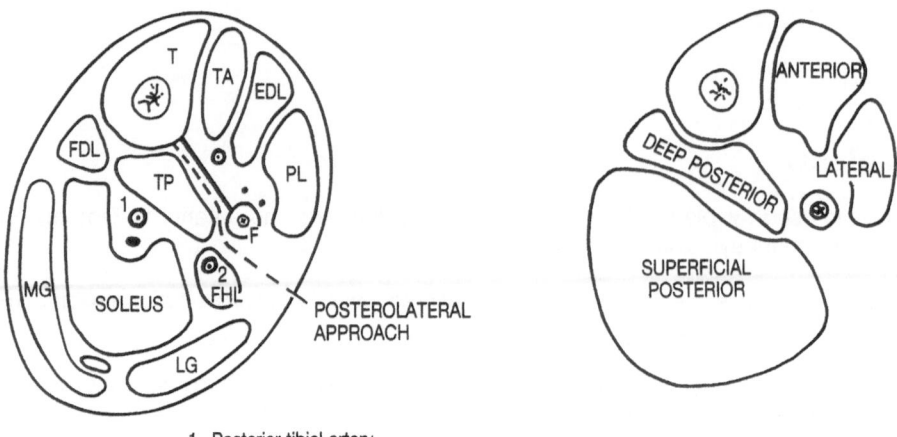

1. Posterior tibial artery
2. Peroneal artery

Fig. b. Transverse section through the middle of the calf.

Fig. c. The compartments of the leg.

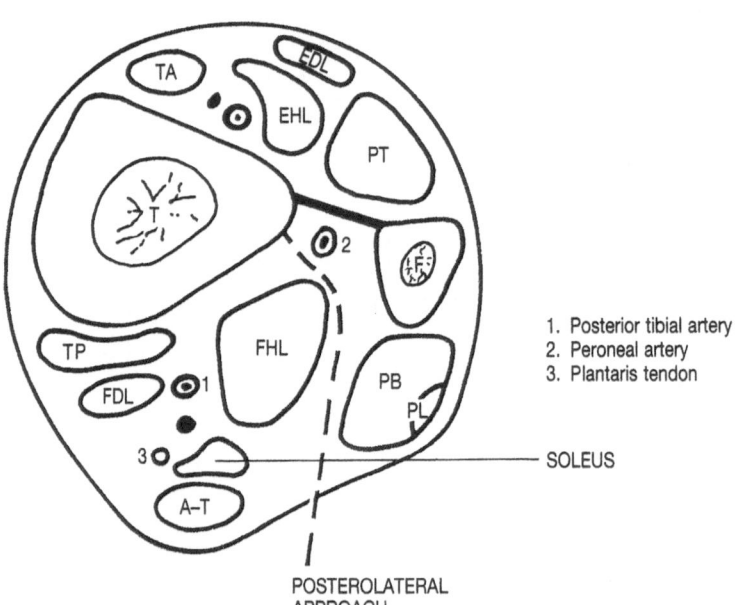

1. Posterior tibial artery
2. Peroneal artery
3. Plantaris tendon

Fig. d. Transverse section proximal to ankle.

Posterior

This is used for plating a tibial nonunion when the skin anteriorly is of doubtful viability. It can also be used to decompress the deep and superficial posterior compartments in compartment syndrome (Figs. b and c).

- The posterolateral approach is the safest.

- Incise the skin along the lateral aspect of the gastrocnemius.

- Develop the plane between gastrocsoleus and the flexor hallucis longus posteriorly and the peroneal muscles anteriorly (Figs. b and d).

- Expose the posterior surface of the fibula and dissect tibialis posterior from the intermuscular septum. Strip the muscle subperiosteally to expose the posterior surface of the tibia.

- The posterior tibial nerve is protected by the FHL and tibialis posterior.

- The peroneal nerves are protected by the fibula.

- The anterior tibial vessels are protected by the interosseous membrane.

Approaches to the Ankle

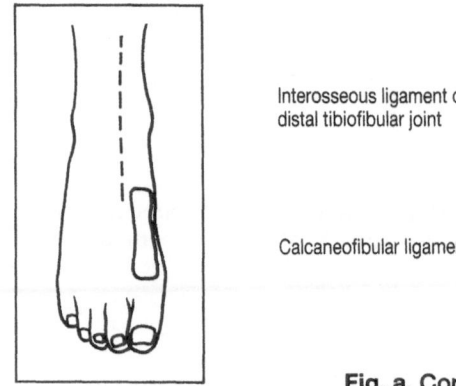

Interosseous ligament of distal tibiofibular joint

TALUS

Deltoid ligament

Calcaneofibular ligament

OS CALCIS

Fig. a. Coronal section of the ankle.

Fig. b. The anterior relations of the ankle.

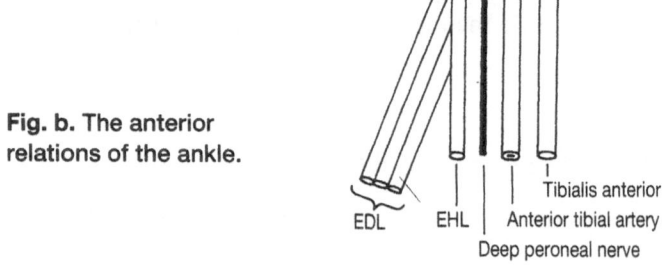

EDL   EHL   Tibialis anterior

Anterior tibial artery

Deep peroneal nerve

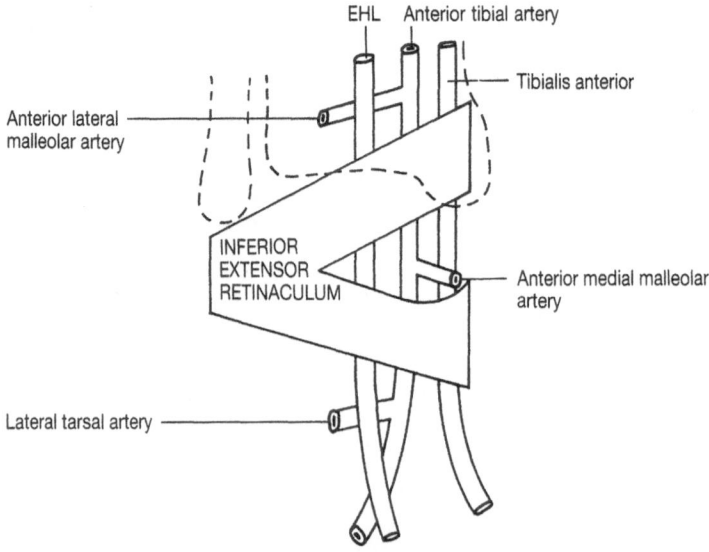

EHL   Anterior tibial artery

Tibialis anterior

Anterior lateral malleolar artery

INFERIOR EXTENSOR RETINACULUM

Anterior medial malleolar artery

Lateral tarsal artery

Fig. c. The relations of the anterior tibial artery.

Fractures around the ankle are very common. The tip of the lateral malleolus lies distal to the tip of the medial malleolus and the whole of the fibula lies slightly posterior to the tibia (Fig. a). The posterior edge of the distal tibia is often called the posterior malleolus.

The medial and lateral malleoli lie immediately under the skin but it is better to expose them through an incision placed over the adjacent soft tissue.

The ankle may be opened to remove loose bodies, for arthrodesis, or for reconstruction of severe fractures. The tarsus is most commonly exposed for arthrodesis.

Anterior

The approach is (Fig. b):

either 1. between the extensor hallucis longus tendon and the extensor digitorum longus tendons retracting the neurovascular bundle medially,

or   2. between the extensor hallucis longus tendon and the tibialis anterior tendon retracting the neurovascular bundle laterally.

- After dividing the extensor retinaculum mobilise the anterior tibial artery by dividing the anterior lateral malleolar and lateral tarsal arteries if it is to be retracted medially, or the anterior medial malleolar artery if it is to be retracted laterally (Fig. c).

- Open the joint by incising its capsule.

Approaches to the Ankle (continued)

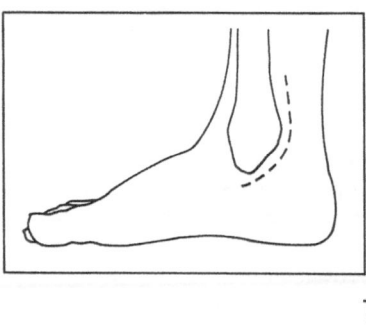

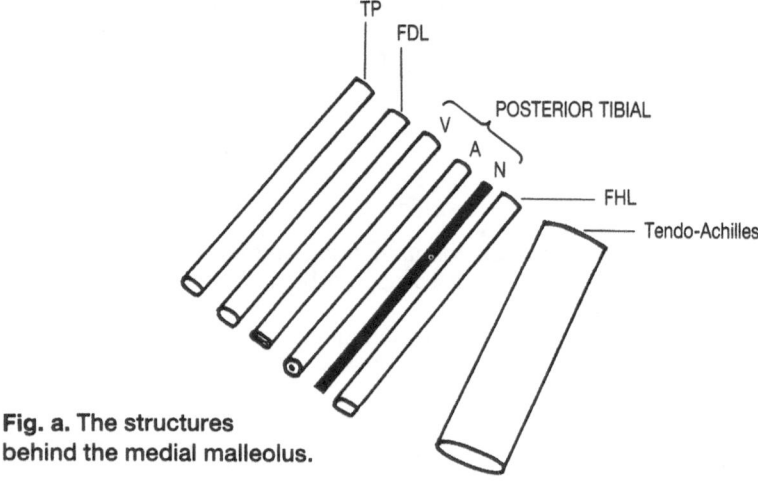

Fig. a. The structures behind the medial malleolus.

TP
FDL
POSTERIOR TIBIAL
V
A
N
FHL
Tendo-Achilles

Fig. b. Medial view of the ankle.

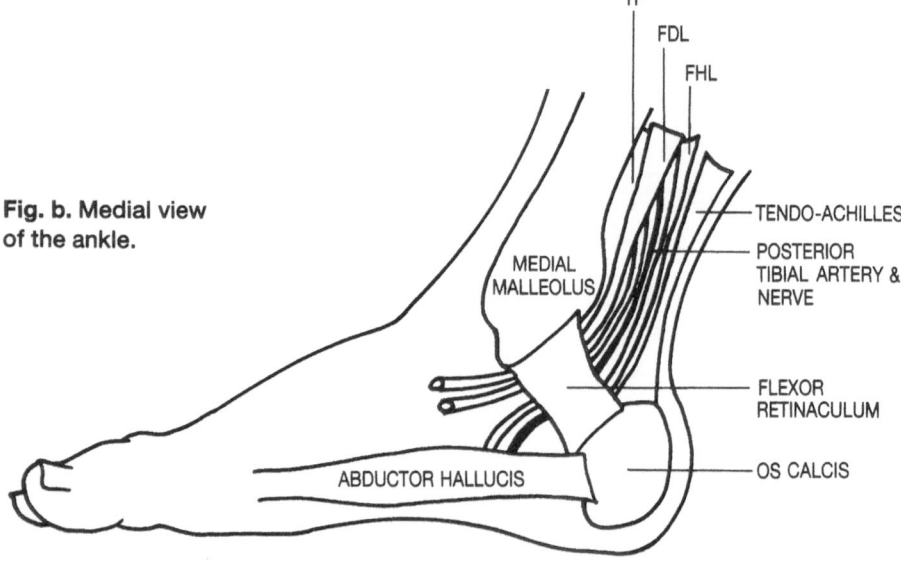

TP
FDL
FHL
TENDO-ACHILLES
POSTERIOR TIBIAL ARTERY & NERVE
MEDIAL MALLEOLUS
FLEXOR RETINACULUM
OS CALCIS
ABDUCTOR HALLUCIS

Medial

This approach exposes important structures. It can be used to approach the posterior malleolus, for posteromedial release for talipes equinovarus, and for exposing the posterior tibial nerve in tarsal tunnel syndrome.

- Divide the retinaculum and deepen the wound between tibialis posterior and flexor digitorum longus anteriorly and the flexor hallucis longus and the neurovascular bundle posteriorly (Figs. a and b).

- To expose the branches of the posterior tibial nerve, detach the origin of the abductor hallucis from the os calcis. Identify and coagulate the calcaneal branches of the posterior tibial vessels which enter the inner surface of the muscle.

Anterolateral Approach to the Tarsus

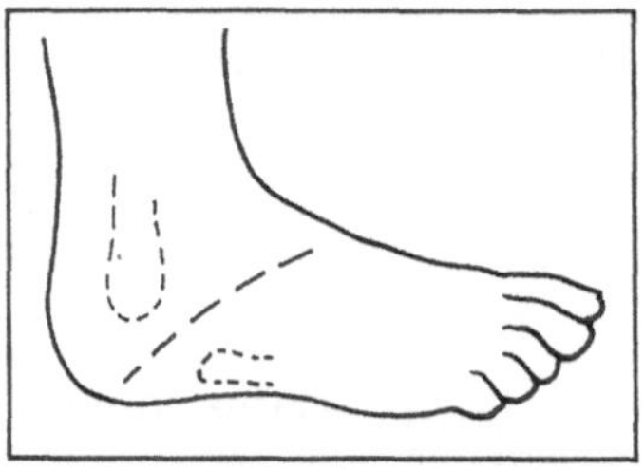

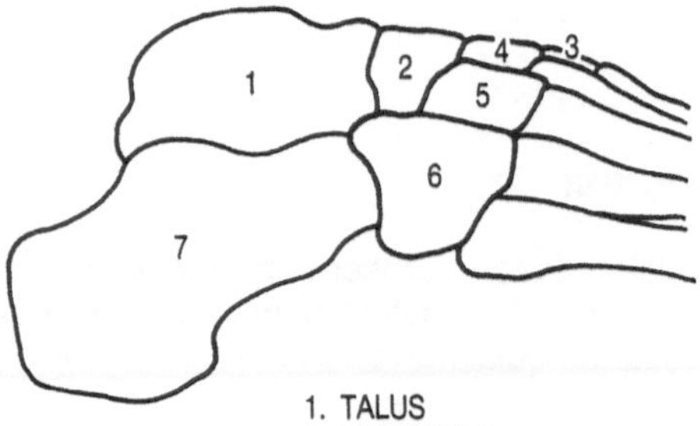

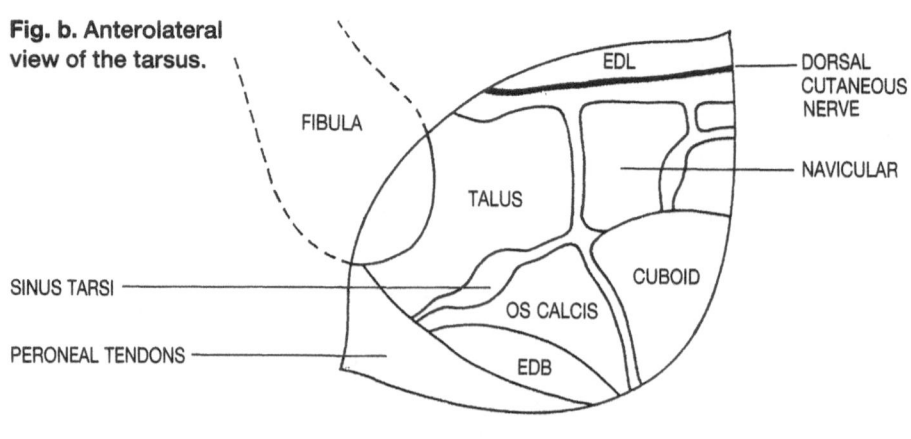

1. TALUS
2. NAVICULAR
3. MEDIAL CUNEIFORM
4. INTERMEDIATE CUNEIFORM
5. LATERAL CUNEIFORM
6. CUBOID
7. OS CALCIS (CALCANEUS)

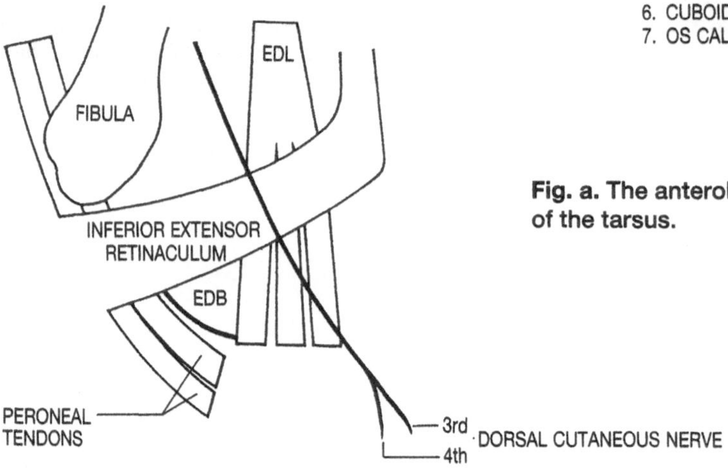

EDL

FIBULA

INFERIOR EXTENSOR
RETINACULUM

EDB

PERONEAL
TENDONS

3rd
4th · DORSAL CUTANEOUS NERVE

Fig. a. The anterolateral relations
of the tarsus.

Fig. b. Anterolateral
view of the tarsus.

FIBULA

EDL

DORSAL
CUTANEOUS
NERVE

NAVICULAR

TALUS

SINUS TARSI

CUBOID

OS CALCIS

PERONEAL TENDONS

EDB

Anterolateral Approach to the Tarsus

This approach is commonly used to perform a triple arthrodesis; calcaneocuboid, subtalar, and talo navicular fusion.

- Incise the skin from the talo navicular joint to 2.5 cm distal to the fibula.

- Identify the dorsal cutaneous branch of the superficial peroneal nerve, the inferior border of the extensor retinaculum, and the lateral border of the peroneus tertius tendon (Fig. a).

- Incise the lower border of the extensor retinaculum transversely to expose the extensor digitorum brevis muscle. Preserve the sensory nerve.

- Dissect the extensor digitorum brevis from the floor of the sinus tarsi (the tunnel between the posterior and middle facets of the subtalar joint) (Fig. b).

- Remove the soft tissue from the sinus tarsi to expose the subtalar, calcaneocuboid, and talo navicular joints.

- Open the joints by incising their capsules.

Approaches to the Forefoot and Toes

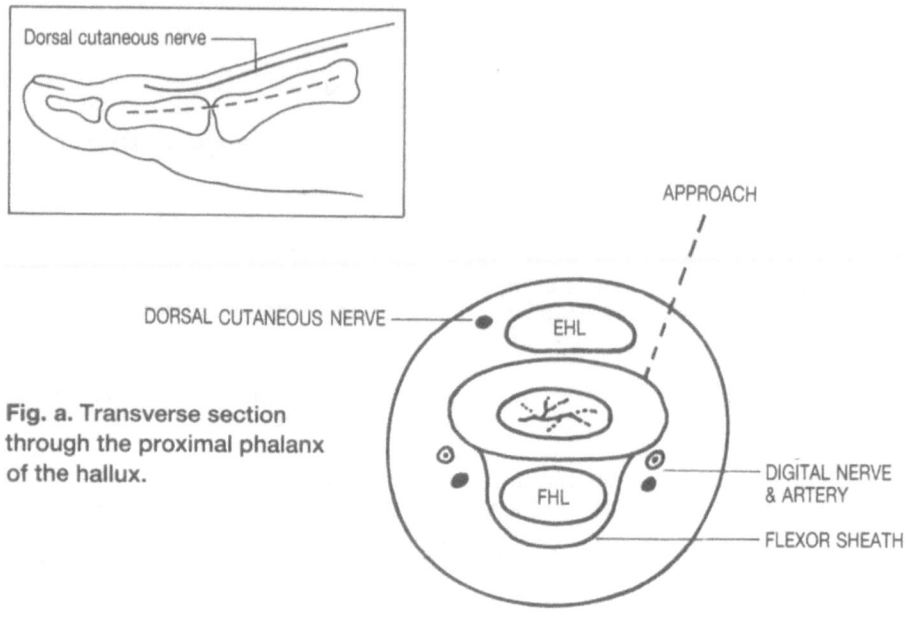

Dorsal cutaneous nerve

APPROACH

DORSAL CUTANEOUS NERVE — EHL

Fig. a. Transverse section through the proximal phalanx of the hallux.

DIGITAL NERVE & ARTERY

FHL

FLEXOR SHEATH

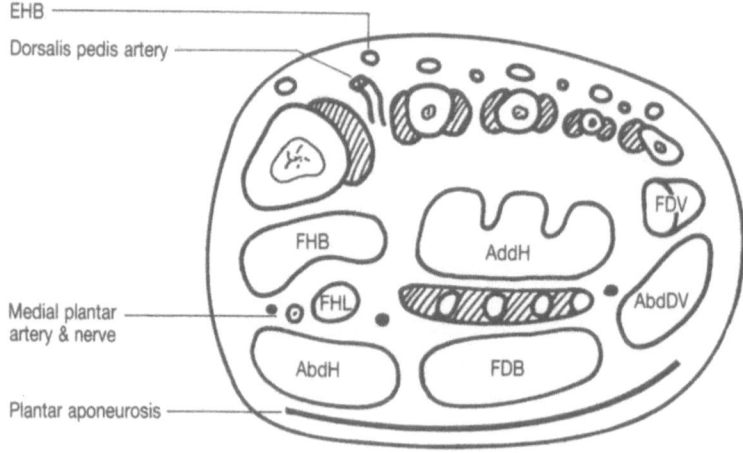

EHB

Dorsalis pedis artery

FDV

FHB

AddH

Medial plantar artery & nerve

FHL

AbdDV

AbdH

FDB

Plantar aponeurosis

4th layer   Interossei
3rd layer   Flexor hallucis brevis, adductor hallucis, flexor
            digiti quinti
2nd layer   Flexor hallucis longus, flexor digitorum longus,
            lumbricals
1st layer   Abductor hallucis, flexor digitorum brevis, abductor
            digiti quinti

Fig. b. Transverse section through the base of the metatarsals.

The forefoot and toes have analogous anatomy to the hand and fingers, but are modified for bipedal gait.

Dorsal

The extensor tendons, metacarpals, and phalanges are exposed by longitudinal incisions placed directly over the required site. To reach two adjacent metatarsals place a single longitudinal incision between them.

Approach to the 1st MTP joint

This approach is used for all operations on this joint including those for bunionectomy, hallux valgus, and hallux rigidus.

- Place the incision on the dorsum of the toe medial to the tendon of extensor hallucis longus, to avoid the dorsal cutaneous branch of the superficial peroneal nerve (Fig. a).

- Deepen the wound just medial to the extensor tendon dividing periosteum and capsule (Fig. b).

Approaches to the Forefoot and Toes (continued)

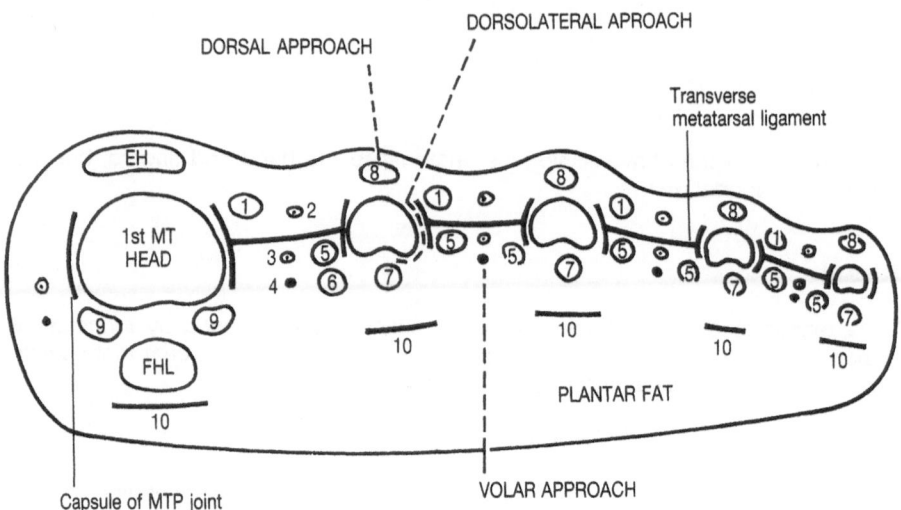

1. Dorsal interosseous tendon
2. Dorsal metatarsal artery
3. Plantar metatarsal artery
4. Plantar digital nerve
5. Plantar interosseous tendon
6. Lumbrical
7. Flexor digitorum tendon
8. Extensor digitorum tendon
9. Sesamoid
10. Plantar aponeurosis

Fig. c. Transverse section through the metatarsal heads.

Dorsolateral Approach to Flexor Tendons

This is used in mobile clawing of the toes, where the flexor tendons are relatively short, and may be simply divided or the long flexor may be transferred to the extensor tendon.

- Make a longitudinal incision on the lateral side of the extensor tendon in the phalanx.

- Incise to bone and strip the periosteum off the bone round to the volar surface. This protects the neurovascular bundle, and exposes the flexor tendons (Fig. c).

Volar

This is used to explore the space between the metatarsal heads in Morton's neuroma or intermetatarsal bursitis.

- Make a longitudinal incision through the sole directly under the affected cleft.

- Incise and reflect the plantar fat dividing the transverse fascial bands (Fig. c).

- Expose the plantar digital nerve, between the metatarsal heads, and trace it distally till it divides into its two phalangeal branches.

III. Spine

Approaches to the Cervical Spine

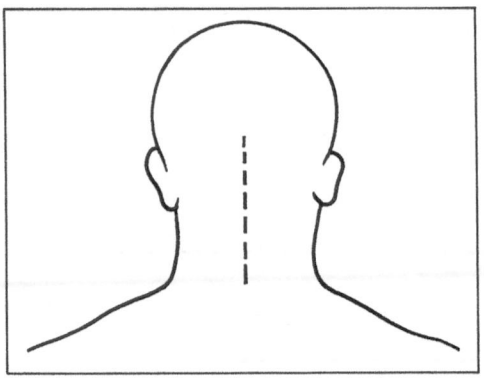

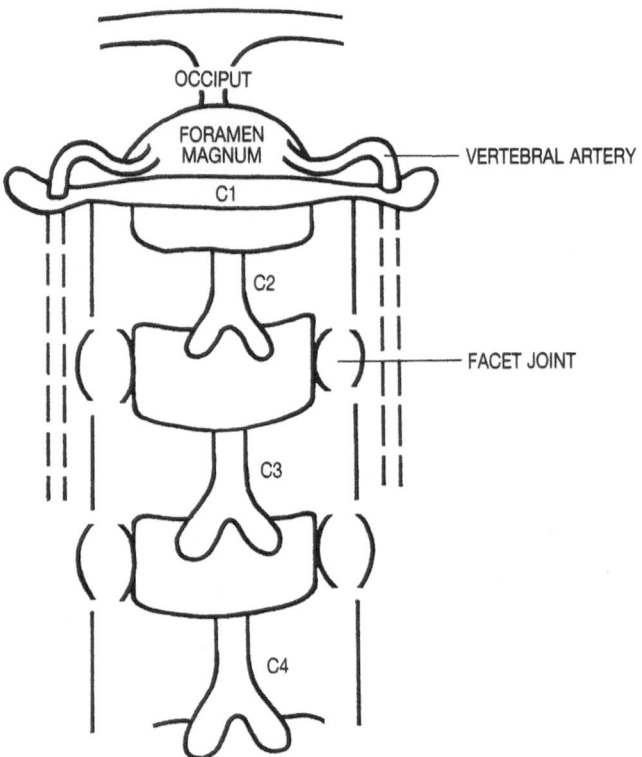

Fig. a. Posterior approach to the upper cervical spine.

Posterior

This approach is used to stabilise the cervical spine in the presence of instability from trauma, tumour or rheumatoid arthritis. It is approached by a direct midline incision.

- Strip the paraspinal muscles carefully from the spinous processes and laminae, and from the occiput.

- Avoid damage to the vertebral artery as it enters the foramen magnum and also as it ascends lateral to the facet joints (Fig. a).

Approaches to the Cervical Spine (continued)

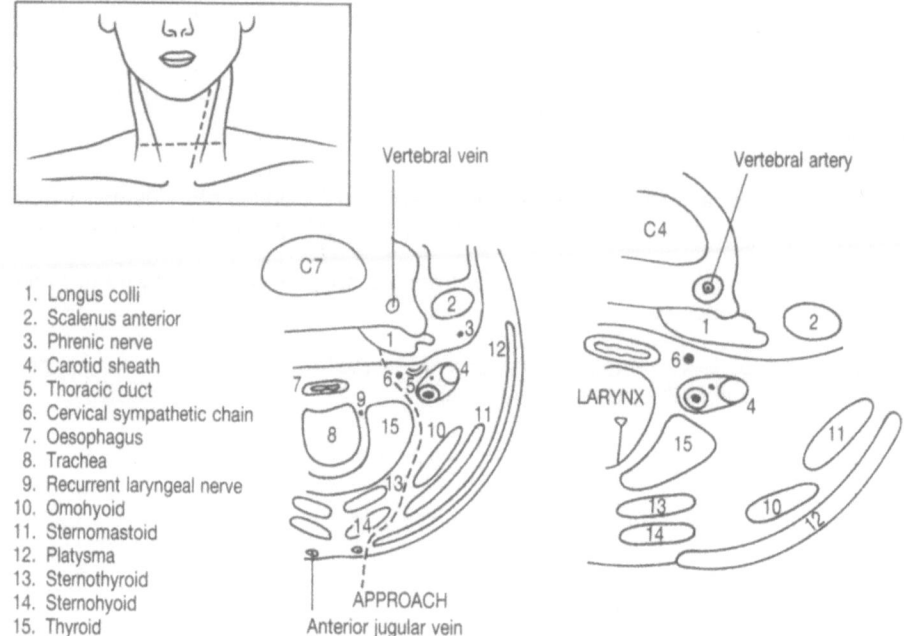

1. Longus colli
2. Scalenus anterior
3. Phrenic nerve
4. Carotid sheath
5. Thoracic duct
6. Cervical sympathetic chain
7. Oesophagus
8. Trachea
9. Recurrent laryngeal nerve
10. Omohyoid
11. Sternomastoid
12. Platysma
13. Sternothyroid
14. Sternohyoid
15. Thyroid

Vertebral vein

C7

Vertebral artery

C4

LARYNX

APPROACH
Anterior jugular vein

Fig. a. Transverse section through C7.

Fig. b. Transverse section through C4.

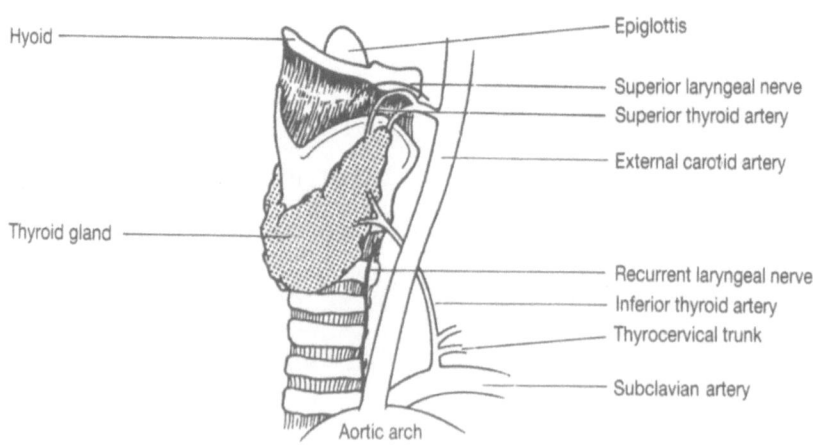

Hyoid

Thyroid gland

Aortic arch

Epiglottis

Superior laryngeal nerve
Superior thyroid artery

External carotid artery

Recurrent laryngeal nerve
Inferior thyroid artery
Thyrocervical trunk

Subclavian artery

Fig. c. Lateral view of the structures of the neck.

Anterior

C3 to C7 can be exposed by a transverse incision or an incision along the anterior border of sternomastoid. The approach can be from either side.

- Avoid damaging the anterior jugular veins on deepening the incision (Figs. a and b).

- The approach is via the anterior border of the sternomastoid muscle. Divide the omohyoid. Retract sternomastoid laterally and the strap muscles medially.

- Identify the carotid sheath and retract it laterally, if necessary dividing the superior thyroid vessels, and middle thyroid vein (Fig. c).

- Retract the oesophagus, trachea or larynx, and the thyroid with the recurrent laryngeal nerve in the opposite direction to reveal the vertebral bodies.

- Avoid damage to the recurrent laryngeal nerve, the phrenic nerve as it lies on scalenus anterior, and on the left, at the level of C7, the thoracic duct.

- Incise the prevertebral fascia in the midline and retract it medially and laterally avoiding damage to the cervical sympathetic chain, the vertebral artery (before it enters the vertebral foramina at C6) and the vascular longus colli muscles.

- Separate the longus colli muscles from the discs and vertebral bodies. Nutrient vessels between muscle and bone may bleed at this stage.

Approaches to the Thoracic Spine

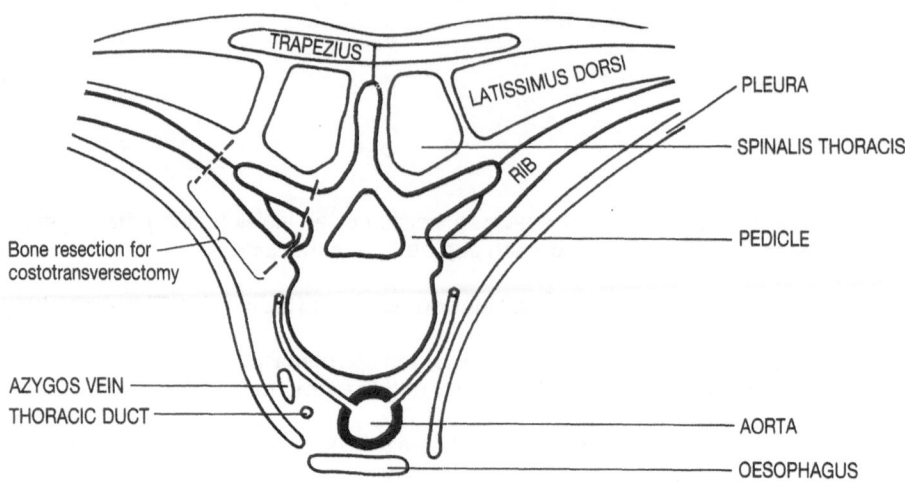

Fig. a. Transverse section through T7.

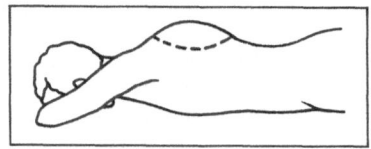

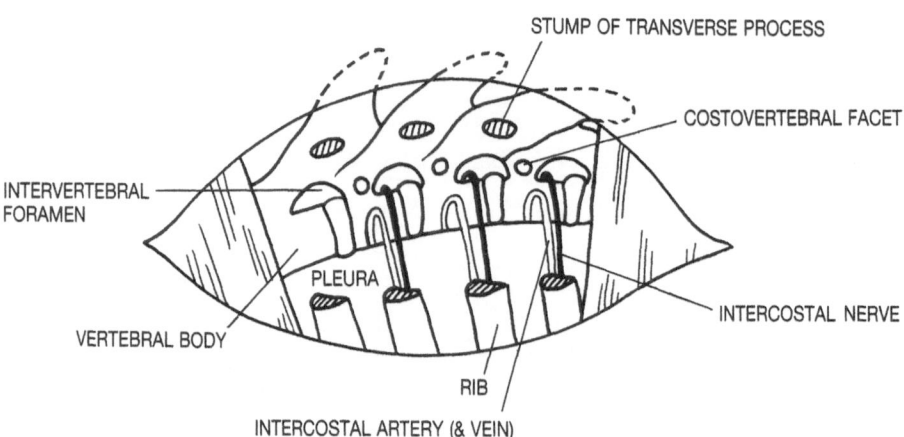

Fig. b. Posterolateral exposure of the thoracic spine.

Approaches to the Thoracic Spine

Transthoracic

A thoracotomy is performed usually through the left side as the aorta tolerates handling better than the vena cava. The level is two ribs above the vertebral body to be exposed. The rib is resected for better exposure.

- The thoracic duct lies to the right of the oesophagus in the lower posterior mediastinum crossing behind the oesophagus at T5 (Fig. a).

- The intercostal vessels traverse the waists of the vertebral bodies.

Posterolateral

In tuberculous abscesses the paravertebral space can be drained via a costotransversectomy (Fig. a).

- Place the patient in the prone position.

- Make a longitudinal curved incision convex laterally centred on the kyphos.

- Divide the trapezius and rhomboids longitudinally 3 cm from the midline.

- Strip and display the three ribs at the apex of the kyphos. Divide 5 cm of each rib starting at the costotransverse joint (Fig. a).

- Identify the two adjacent intercostal nerves and trace them medially as far as the intervertebral foramina, dividing the transverse process to gain access (Fig. b).

- Divide the pedicle if the spinal canal is to be explored (Fig. a).

Approaches to the Lumbar Spine

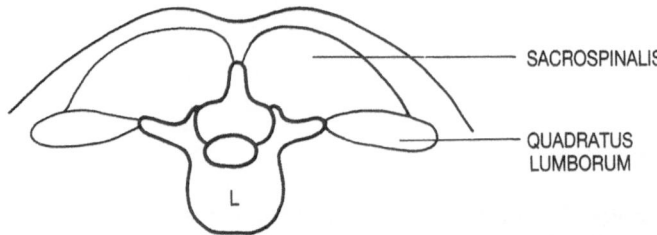

SACROSPINALIS

QUADRATUS LUMBORUM

L

Fig. a. Transverse section through a lumbar vertebra.

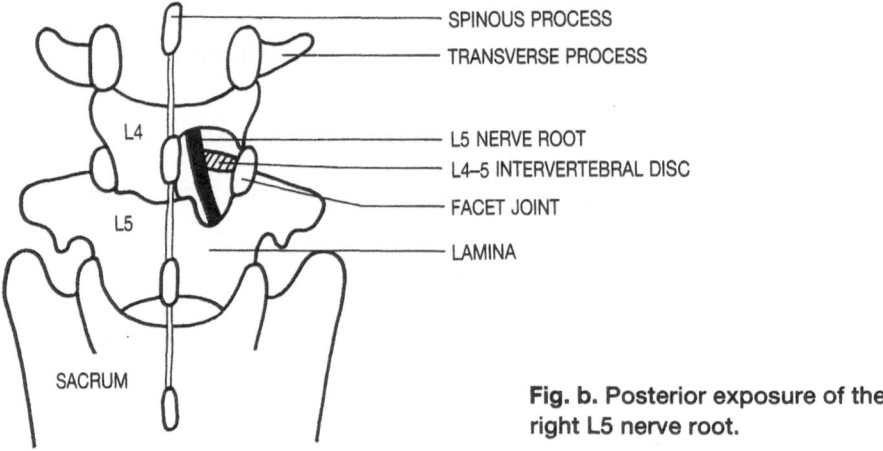

SPINOUS PROCESS

TRANSVERSE PROCESS

L4

L5 NERVE ROOT

L4–5 INTERVERTEBRAL DISC

FACET JOINT

LAMINA

L5

SACRUM

Fig. b. Posterior exposure of the right L5 nerve root.

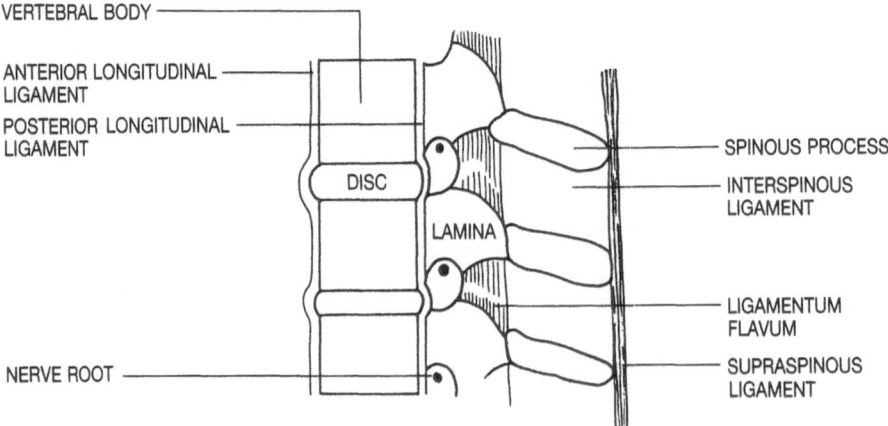

VERTEBRAL BODY

ANTERIOR LONGITUDINAL LIGAMENT

POSTERIOR LONGITUDINAL LIGAMENT

DISC

LAMINA

NERVE ROOT

SPINOUS PROCESS

INTERSPINOUS LIGAMENT

LIGAMENTUM FLAVUM

SUPRASPINOUS LIGAMENT

Fig. c. Sagittal section through the lumbar spine.

Approaches to the Lumbar Spine

Posterior

Access to the posterior aspect of the vertebral column is required for the removal of protruding intervertebral discs, spinal fusion, and the correction of scoliosis.

The L4 nerve root is trapped by the L3/L4 disc before it sweeps round the pedicle of L4 and passes laterally through the root canal. Its main action is knee extension via quadriceps and it supplies sensation around the knee. Damage to it therefore results in loss of the knee reflex. The L5 nerve root is trapped by the L4/L5 disc. Its main action is extension of the great toe. It supplies sensation down the outer side of the calf and dorsum of the foot to the great toe. The S1 nerve root is trapped by the L5/S1 disc. Its main action is to dorsiflex the ankle via the calf muscles and it supplies sensation to the sole and the outer border of the foot. Damage to it therefore results in loss of the ankle reflex. This allows clinical assessment of the level to be explored, and is confirmed by radiological investigation.

- The patient is placed prone or on the side with the lumbar spine flexed. Identify the level of the disc. The spinous processes between L5 and S1 can fit the thumb, and between L4 and L5 the index finger.

- Expose the required level by a midline incision along the tips of the spinous processes. Strip the paraspinal muscles from the spinous processes and the laminae laterally to the facet joints and for spinal fusion further laterally to the tips of the transverse processes (Figs. a and b).

- Confirm the level to be explored by identifying L5/S1. It is the lowermost mobile level, the sacrum sounds dull to percussion, and the lower border of the L5 lamina is sharp.

- To excise a disc perform a fenestration on the correct side. Nibble the inferior part of the lamina since the ligamentum flavum is attached to its superior border (Figs. b and c).

- To decompress the spinal canal, e.g. for spinal stenosis, excise the spinous process and laminae (laminectomy).

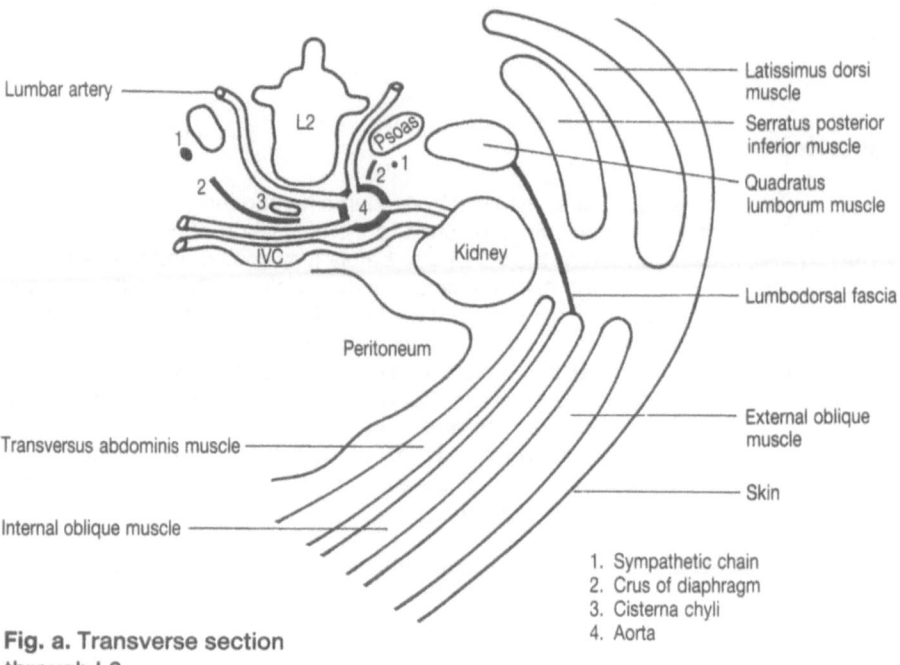

Lumbar artery

L2

Psoas

1
2
3
IVC
4
2 •1

Kidney

Latissimus dorsi muscle

Serratus posterior inferior muscle

Quadratus lumborum muscle

Lumbodorsal fascia

Peritoneum

External oblique muscle

Skin

Transversus abdominis muscle

Internal oblique muscle

1. Sympathetic chain
2. Crus of diaphragm
3. Cisterna chyli
4. Aorta

Fig. a. Transverse section through L2.

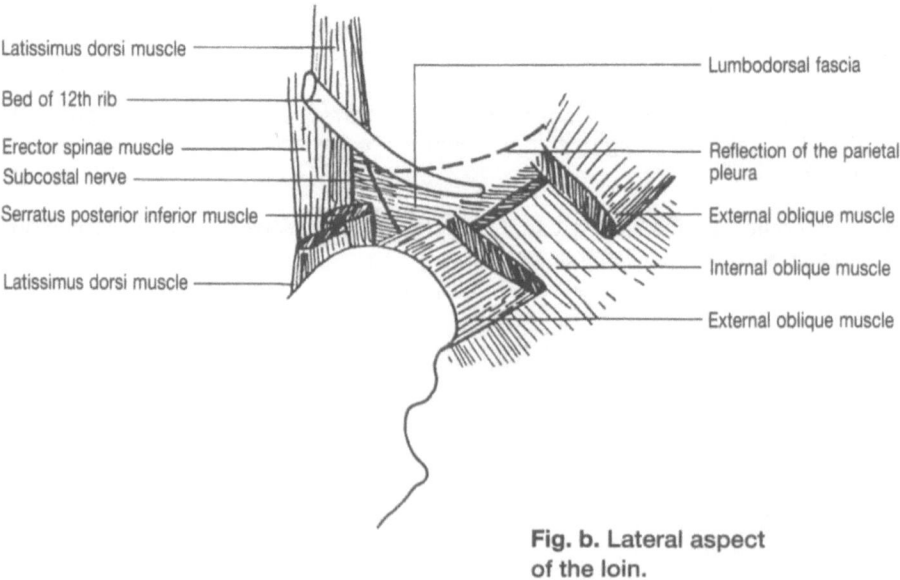

Latissimus dorsi muscle

Bed of 12th rib

Erector spinae muscle

Subcostal nerve

Serratus posterior inferior muscle

Latissimus dorsi muscle

Lumbodorsal fascia

Reflection of the parietal pleura

External oblique muscle

Internal oblique muscle

External oblique muscle

Fig. b. Lateral aspect of the loin.

Anterior

Exposure from T10 to L2 requires resection of the 10th rib.

- The diaphragm is difficult to identify as a separate structure as it approximates to the thoracic cage. Beware damaging the lung as the diaphragm and pleura are divided.

- Expose the thoracolumbar junction by reflecting the diaphragm off the ribs and the crus off the spine (Fig. c page 84).

Exposure of the upper lumbar vertebrae is via a nephrectomy incision using a transcostal or subcostal route.

Subcostal

- The incision extends from the angle of the 12th rib and the anterior border of the erector spinae muscles, and passes forwards 1 cm below and parallel to the 12th rib to a point 2 cm above the anterior superior iliac spine.

- The fibres of the external oblique muscle run in the line of the incision anteriorly with latissimus dorsi, forming the superficial muscle layer at the posterior end of the wound.

- The serratus posterior inferior muscle lies deep to latissimus dorsi. Divide the serratus posterior inferior to expose the lateral edge of the erector spinae and lumbodorsal fascia. Preserve the subcostal nerve as it lies deep to the lumbodorsal fascia (Fig. b).

- Divide the internal oblique and lumbodorsal fascia to enter the perinephric space. Reflect the kidney forwards off the quadratus lumborum muscle.

- The crus of the diaphragm extends distally and ties the aorta to the vertebral bodies (Fig. a opposite and Fig. c, page 84).

- Incise the periosteum over the vertebral body and reflect this, the anterior vertebral ligament and the crus to expose the bone. Isolate the lumbar vessels as they lie in the waist of the vertebral body.

Transcostal

- Incise along the line of the 12th rib dividing the serratus posterior inferior and the latissimus dorsi muscles (Fig. a).

- Resect the 12th rib after incising the periosteum taking care not to damage the pleura.

- Divide the lumbodorsal fascia to gain entry to the perinephric space (Figs. a and b).

Approaches to the Lumbar Spine (continued)

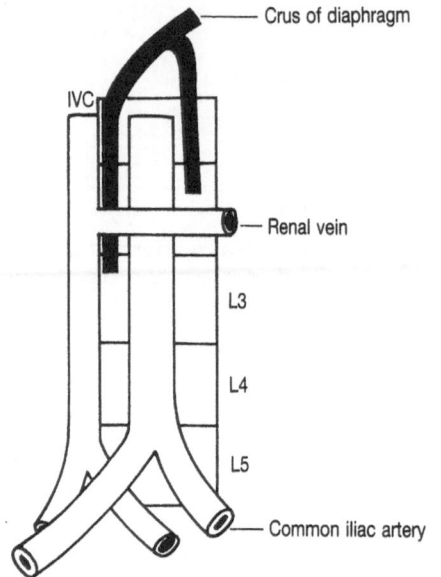

Crus of diaphragm

IVC

Renal vein

L3

L4

L5

Common iliac artery

Fig. c. The relationship of the lumbar spine to the great vessels.

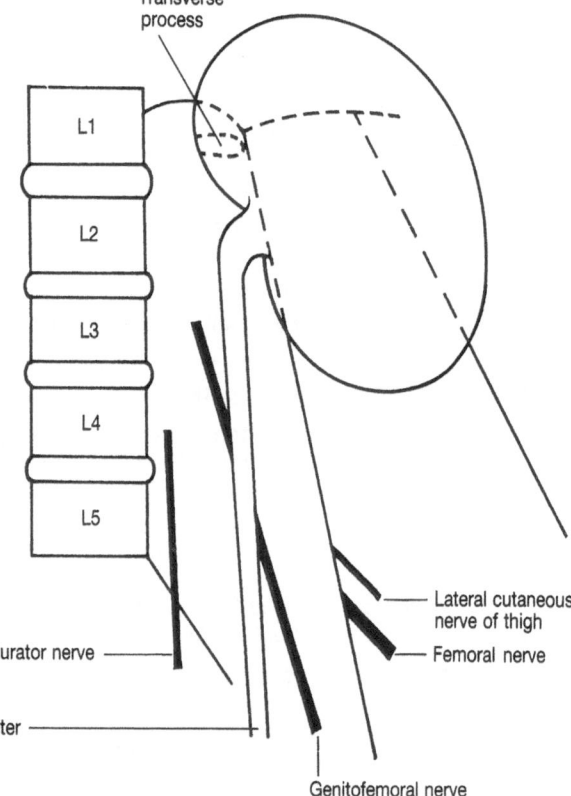

Transverse process

L1

L2

L3

L4

L5

Fig. d. Structures of the posterior abdominal wall.

Obturator nerve

Ureter

Lateral cutaneous nerve of thigh

Femoral nerve

Genitofemoral nerve

Anterolateral Extraperitoneal

This gains access from L3 to lumbosacral junction. The vertebral bodies are approached from the left.

- Make an oblique incision from the tip of the 12th rib extending into the iliac fossa midway between the anterior superior iliac spine and the umbilicus. Deepen the wound to the extraperitoneal space via a gridiron muscle spitting approach and sweep the peritoneum anteriorly.

- Identify the ureter attached to the parietal peritoneum anteriorly to avoid injuring it (Fig. d).

- Identify the genitofemoral nerve lying on iliopsoas (Fig. d).

- Identify and retract the aorta and common iliac vessels to expose the vertebral column. Avoid damage to the sympathetic chain.

- Divide the lumbar fascia taking care to identify, and ligate the relevant segmental lumbar vessels.

Approach to the Sacrum

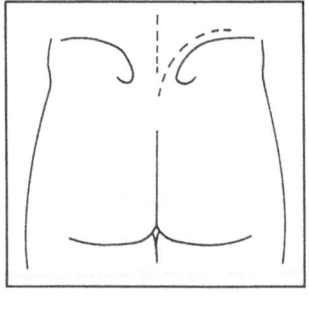

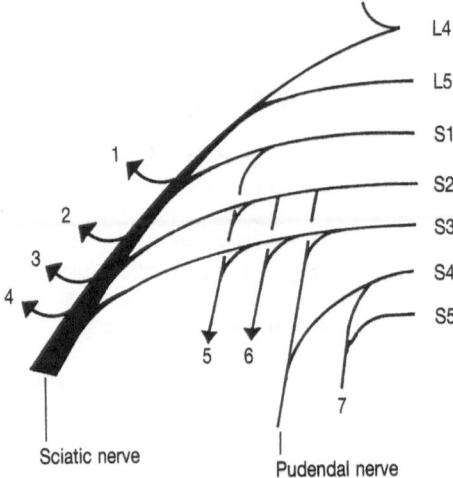

Fig. a. The sacral plexus.

L4
L5
S1
S2
S3
S4
S5

1
2
3
4
5 6
7

Sciatic nerve

Pudendal nerve

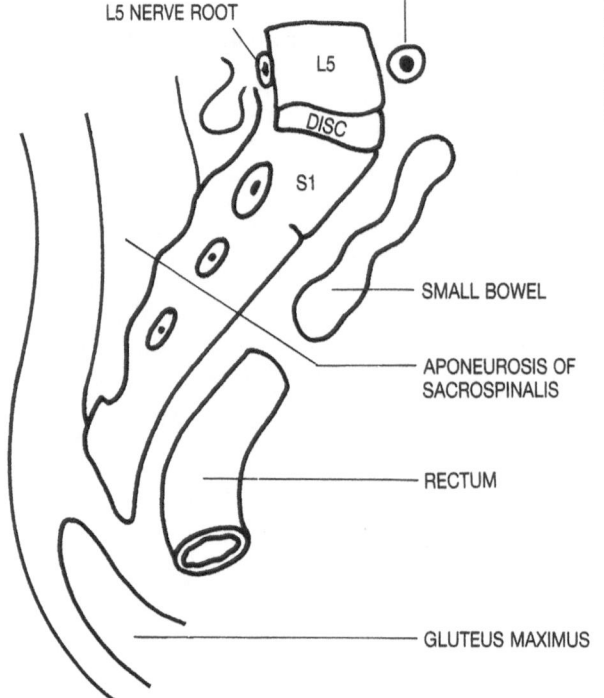

COMMON ILIAC ARTERY

L5 NERVE ROOT

L5

DISC

S1

SMALL BOWEL

APONEUROSIS OF
SACROSPINALIS

RECTUM

GLUTEUS MAXIMUS

1. Superior gluteal nerve
2. Inferior gluteal nerve
3. Nerve to quadratus femoris
4. Nerve to obturator internus
5. Posterior cutaneous nerve of thigh
6. Perforating cutaneous nerve
7. Coccygeal nerve

Fig. b. Parasagittal section of the sacrum.

The roots of the sacral plexus emerge through the anterior sacral foramina to unite in front of piriformis (Fig. a). Branches supply the pelvic muscles, the muscles of the hip, and the skin at the back of the buttock and thigh. It finishes as two main branches; the pudendal nerve, and the sciatic nerve. The pudendal nerve (S 2, 3, 4) innervates the perineum and particularly the external urethral sphincter. If divided bilaterally it leads to incontinence. In sacral resection for chordoma the S4 and S5 nerve roots are sacrificed but the others are preserved to keep bladder function. The sciatic nerve innervates the knee flexors and the muscles below the knee and supplies sensation to the sole of the foot and the back of the calf.

The sacral plexus may be damaged by fractures of the sacrum or tumours. The sacro-iliac joint may be affected by infections or disrupted in severe pelvic injuries.

Posterior Approach

- Place the patient prone. Make a midline incision along the spinous processes.

- Reflect the aponeurosis of sacrospinalis laterally (Fig. b).

- In sacral resection, excise the coccyx and mobilise the rectum, detach gluteus maximus, piriformis, coccygeus, the sacrotuberous and sacrospinous ligaments, and divide the S4 and S5 roots. Remove the sacrum preserving the S1, S2, and S3 roots at least on one side.

Approaches to the Sacro-Iliac Joint

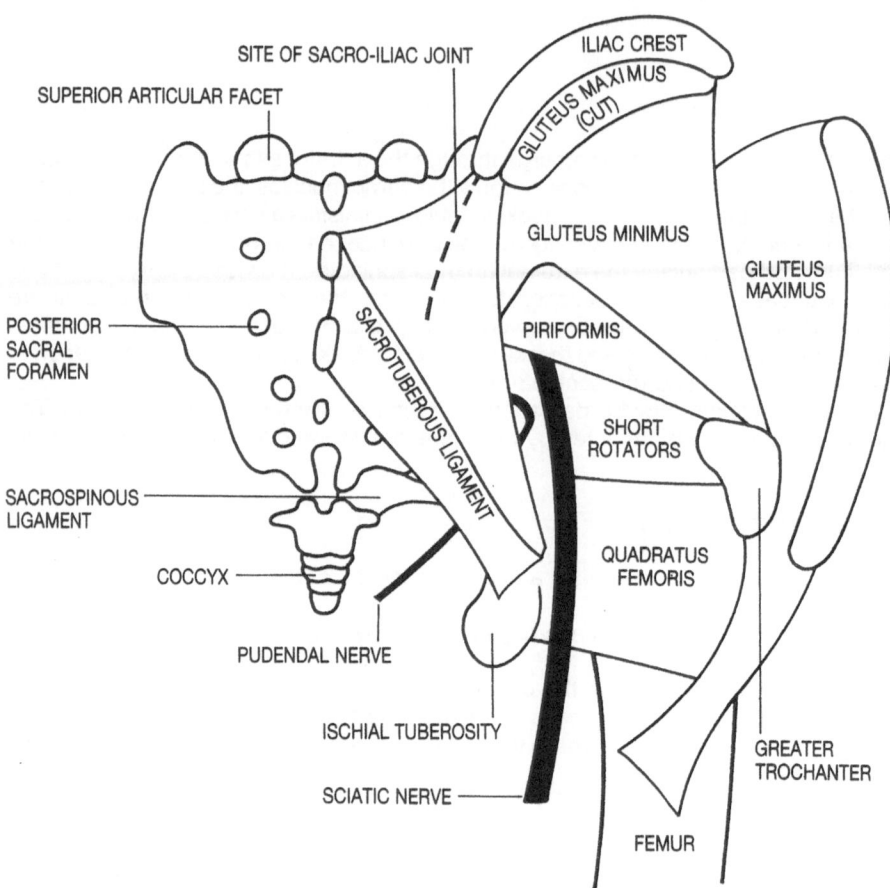

Fig. a. Posterior view of the
sacrum and buttock.

Approaches to the Sacro-Iliac Joint

Posterior

- Make a curved incision along the iliac crest to the midline of the sacrum.

- Detach gluteus maximus from the iliac crest, and the sacrotuberous ligament from the iliac crest and the sacrum (Fig. a).

- To expose the joint excise a 2 cm strip of the ilium from the posterior superior iliac spine to the posterior inferior iliac spine.

Anterior

- Detach the abdominal muscles from the iliac crest.

- Strip iliacus subperiosteally from the inner side of the iliac wing. Palpate the joint and expose it by detaching the anterior sacro-iliac ligament.

Appendix

Suggested Further Reading

Campbell's Operative Orthopaedics, Crenshaw AH (ed), CV Mosby Co, 1987
Cunningham's Textbook of Anatomy, Romanes GJ (ed), Oxford University Press, 1972
Gray's Anatomy, Warwick R and Williams PL (eds), Longman, 1973
Operative Surgery, Rob C and Smith R (eds), Butterworth and Co, 1979